In Search of Nursing Science

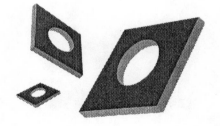

In Search of Nursing Science

Edited by **Anna Omery**
Christine E. Kasper
Gayle G. Page

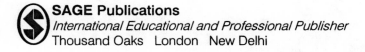
SAGE Publications
International Educational and Professional Publisher
Thousand Oaks   London   New Delhi

For information address:

SAGE Publications, Inc.
2455 Teller Road
Thousand Oaks, California 91320
E-mail: order@sagepub.com

SAGE Publications Ltd.
6 Bonhill Street
London EC2A 4PU
United Kingdom

SAGE Publications India Pvt. Ltd.
M-32 Market
Greater Kailash I
New Delhi 110 048 India

Printed in the United States of America

Library of Congress Cataloging-in-Publication Data

In search of nursing science / edited by Anna Omery, Christine E.
    Kasper, Gayle G. Page.
      p. cm.
    Includes bibliographical references and index.
    ISBN 0-8039-5093-4 (cl). — ISBN 0-8039- 5094-2 (pbk.: alk. paper)
    1. Nursing—Philosophy. 2. Science—Philosophy. I. Omery, Anna.
II. Kasper, Christine E. III. Page, Gayle G.
    [DNLM: 1. Philosophy, Nursing. 2. Science. WY 86 I35 1995]
RT86.5.I5 1995
610.73'01—dc20   94-37207
DNLM/DLC

This book is printed on acid free paper.

             00 01 02 03 9 8 7 6 5

Sage Production Editor: Diane S. Foster

Contents

Preface   ix

Section I: Introduction and the Empiricist School of Thought   1

1. Introduction: Nursing Science for Nursing Practice   3
   Sue Karen Donaldson

2. Contemporary Empiricism   13
   Sandra J. Weiss

3. Pragmatism: The Problem With the Bottom Line   27
   Christine E. Kasper

Section II: Revolutionary/Evolutionary Philosophy of Science   41

4. Science as Tradition and Tradition Shattering:
   Thomas Kuhn's Philosophy of Science   43
   Jacquelyn Ann K. Kegley

5. Moving Beyond: A Generative Philosophy of Science   58
   *Barbara Riegel, Anna Omery, Evelyn Calvillo, Naiema Gaber
   Elsayed, Patricia Lee, Pamela Shuler,* and *Bonnie Ellen Siegel*

6. Science as Problem Solving   72
   Sara T. Fry

7. An Evolutionary Approach to the Discipline
   of Nursing and Nursing Administration   81
   Cathy Rodgers Ward

Section III: Postmodern Philosophy of Science   91

8. Feminism, Science, and Nursing   93
   Ruth Ginzberg

9. The Method Question   106
   Sandra Harding

10. Pain: An Issue of Gender   127
    Gayle Giboney Page

11. Phenomenology and Science   139
    Anna Omery and Carol Mack

12. The Experience of Surgery:
    Phenomenological Clinical Nursing Research   159
    Marlene Zichi Cohen

13. A Hermeneutical Human Science for Nursing   175
    Richard H. Steeves and David L. Kahn

14. Passages Through the Heart: A Hermeneutic of Choice   194
    Francelyn Reeder

15. Critical Theory for Science of Nursing Practice   205
    Hesook Suzie Kim and Inger Margrethe Holter

16. Methodology for Critical Theory:
    Critical Action Research   220
    Inger Margrethe Holter and Hesook Suzie Kim

17. Poststructuralist Science: An Historical
    Account of Profound Visibility   233
    Laura Cox Dzurec

18. Severe Mental Disability? Or a Play of Wills?   245
    Laura Cox Dzurec

Section IV: The Relationship Between Science and Practice   261

19. Applied Science, Practice, and Intervention Technology   263
    Anne H. Bishop and John R. Scudder, Jr.

20. Science and Practice: The Nature of Knowledge   275
     Hannah Dean

21. Science as the Predictor of Professional
     Recognition and Success   291
     Luther Christman

Epilogue: The Journey Continues   295

Index   298

About the Contributors   303

Preface

This book began as a quest of its own. It grew out of our personal struggles to identify a specific philosophy of science that was consistent with the discipline of nursing. It quickly became apparent to us, however, that no one specific philosophy seemed adequate. There was no one school of thought that seemed to definitively indicate to us that our journey had been completed, that here in this place, in these ideas, nursing could safely harbor its future knowledge development.

In studying the traditional schools of thought on science, we found insufficiencies. Although there were schools of thought that appealed to each of us as individuals, there was no single school of thought that we could agree on as reflecting nursing. No one belief system seemed to reflect our small group, a group that might be seen as representative of nursing in all of its diversity, for in our group is a phenomenologist, a feminist, and an empiricist—and this is a single individual!

In our journey, we made another discovery that seemed very important to us. We could identify no centralized forum that had as its purpose the comparison of various philosophies of science and how a particular philosophy guides knowledge development; therefore, on our journey we had to embark on as many trails as there were philosophies. Although there was much to wonder at and appreciate in having to take such an extensive journey, it was also frustrating. We longed for a more comprehensive roadway for our exploration. This book is the culmination of our effort to try to build such a roadway for those who are attempting a similar journey.

This does not mean that we wish to keep others from exploring the trails we have explored; rather, the effort here is to assist those embarking on their journey. We desire in this volume to give our novice fellow explorers an easier beginning for their quest, recognizing that the ways to knowledge development will always require sustained effort. For those who are more expert explorers, we hope this volume will provide a vista for their journey, a lookout as it were from which they might review the territory that they have traveled previously and gain some perspective for those regions they have yet to chart.

Before embarking on this trail, we wish to share with our fellow explorers the compass that guided our direction, our aim. What we are attempting to accomplish with *In Search of Nursing Science* is to promote our belief that a plurality of philosophies may be necessary to reflect the many facets of nursing science; that is, no one view may be sufficient to embrace or drive nursing knowledge in its totality. Herein, we provide an anthology of conceptions of Western science in all their diversity. We leave it to our fellow travelers (readers) to ponder which of these competing and often, at least at first glance, incompatible philosophies can or should reflect nursing knowledge. We hope that you, the reader, will be encouraged to think openly and consider each view, including empiricism, pragmatism, paradigmatic, problem solving, feminism, phenomenology, hermeneutics, critical theory, and poststructuralism, for its relevance to the science of nursing.

The book is organized into four sections. The first three explore the different schools of philosophical thought of science currently being debated as the basis in and for nursing knowledge development. The final section concentrates on the possible relationships between science and practice. Our organization is designed so that selected chapters describing a particular view of science are usually followed by companion chapters that are intended to provide the reader with an explication of how that particular view guided nurse scholars in the development of their idea.

In Section I, the Introduction is accompanied by two chapters that explore schools of thought regarding a science that is based in the more traditional empiricist views of science: empiricism and pragmatism. These traditional schools of thought emphasize the view of science as an observable process that results in knowledge that is objective and empirical.

It may be perplexing to some to find no chapter on logical positivism. Our decision to omit such a chapter was deliberate. The limits of this philosophy of science has been well established since the 1960s. Ridiculed as "the Received View," logical positivism has moved beyond its initial tenets and been reformulated within the empiricist tradition. We believe that to present logical positivism as an option, as a possible trail, would lead the traveler to a dead end. For this reason, we have chosen to focus on empiricism and pragmatism, two schools of thought with an origin in positivism. Many of the tenets of empiricism and pragmatism are traditional and bear more than a passing resemblance to positivism. Yet each of these schools has moved beyond the antiquated notions that have limited positivism, and as such, they provide more viable alternates on which to base a belief system for nursing science.

Section I is also the only section in which each chapter does not have a companion chapter providing an example of how the philosophy has been operationalized. The empiricist tradition has been so prevalent in the history of nursing's knowledge development that any work chosen as an example would not necessarily be reflective of the diversity of these traditional philosophical schools of thought in and for nursing and therefore might reflect a more arbitrary decision than we felt comfortable with. As a result, the operationalization of these traditions has been integrated into the chapters describing these philosophies.

Section II focuses on the schools of thought that were the first to challenge the traditional views of science. These schools of thought are classified in this text as revolutionary/evolutionary. Thomas Kuhn's scientific revolution and Larry Laudan's science as problem solving are highlighted in this section.

Section III introduces those schools of thought that are sometimes classified as postmodern. Postmodern thought most directly challenges the objectification of science. The schools presented in this text are feminism, phenomenology, critical theory, and poststructuralism.

The tension that exists in the relationship between science and practice is unique, yet fundamentally critical to professional disciplines such as nursing. Any book exploring the development of knowledge in a professional discipline would be incomplete if these tensions were not addressed. Such is the intent of Section IV. The chapters in this final section explore some of the possible relationships between science and nursing practice.

We wish to acknowledge that this book is not an isolated effort; many other fellow travelers have assisted us. As suggested by Sage, each chapter was internally reviewed by other contributors with expertise in the topic. We also wish to thank Christine Smedley, our editor at Sage, whose patience with us was beyond notable, bordering on the heroic.

We also wish to conclude the beginning with this thought. Knowledge development is always an adventure. For nursing, that adventure has only just begun.

Anna Omery
Christine E. Kasper
Gayle Giboney Page

I

Introduction and the
Empiricist School of Thought

The journey begins with the Introduction. The second and third chapters respectively examine the two current philosophical schools of thought most closely aligned with traditional beliefs in regard to science: empiricism and pragmatism.

In Chapter 1, Sue Donaldson provides an overview of the issues in nursing that drive the development of the discipline and how these issues relate to the many schools of thought delineated in this text. She also sets the context for the discussions that follow in the text.

Donaldson points out that nursing is first and foremost a practice discipline, embodying prescriptive theories. This discipline, nursing, is irrevocably linked to the society it serves, and as a result, its science must address society's needs if its knowledge is to meet the mandate that led to its creation. She concludes by challenging those committed to knowledge development in nursing to always remember that if the discipline of nursing is to thrive then the knowledge of nursing science must fulfill society's mandate. Inherent in this challenge is the premise that any one school of thought, or combination thereof, supporting nursing science will be adequate only if it also supports nursing practice.

Contemporary empiricism is the first philosophical school of thought introduced. Sandra Weiss points outs that major changes in the 1980s and 1990s have occurred in the empirical philosophy of science, such that this belief system has moved away from the antiquated logical positivistic notions that limited its contributions. Weiss differentiates empiricism, its tradition, its tenets, and its possible contributions to important areas of knowledge development in the health sciences.

Pragmatism is the focus of the final chapter of Section I. Christine E. Kasper reviews the origin and structure of pragmatic thought and differentiates pragmatism from empiricism in its focus on the future and outcome. Kasper points out how enticing pragmatism is to a practice discipline; yet she concludes that the danger of pragmatism is that its exclusive use as a philosophy may result in failing to achieve the full range of scientific knowledge required for the discipline of nursing.

Introduction

Nursing Science for Nursing Practice

SUE KAREN DONALDSON

Overview

In its quest for its scientific identity, nursing should heed its motivations. The only defensible reason for the development of the discipline of nursing, which embodies scientific and nonscientific knowledge derived from scholarly inquiry, is to provide knowledge for the professional practice of nursing. But the primary purpose for developing the discipline and the science of nursing is not self-aggrandizement for the profession of nursing. The knowledge of the discipline must ultimately support service to clients and the health of society.

Schools and colleges of nursing were incorporated into institutions of higher education because of the societal value placed on the

AUTHOR'S NOTE: The author thanks Margaret Bull, Ph.D., R.N., for her thoughtful critique and sharing of knowledge of qualitative research.

professional practice of nursing and the recognition that educational programs of a profession are ideally embedded in institutions devoted to scholarly inquiry and research. However, nursing's admittance to higher education was not won because it was a recognized research entity. The discipline and science of nursing continue to be accepted primarily because of the value of professional practice to the end of societal health and not the emerging knowledge structure. This does not diminish the discipline and science of nursing but, rather, puts it in perspective. Furthermore, remaining mindful of the centrality of the professional practice of nursing as the driving force for the development of science of nursing has implications for the nature of the science. The evolutionary passages for nursing leading to its present professional status occurred as a result of tremendous effort on the part of visionary nurse leaders. Upon its first admittance as an independent division of higher education (i.e., schools and colleges of nursing), nursing was recognized almost exclusively as an educational unit. Yet another difficult transition occurred with the establishment of research-based doctoral programs in nursing, in particular the Ph.D. programs; these doctoral degree programs had to be carefully justified at most universities because these degrees redesignated nursing as a research unit associated with a unique discipline.

Throughout the chapter, certain terms are used, as defined here. Practice and clinical practice refer to the professional health-related services of the nurse offered to a client. The client may be either an individual person or a group of people. Given these definitions, the meaning of "clinical practice" can be extrapolated to include professional nursing activities, such as establishment of health policies on behalf of the client, as well as direct client service. Client health problems refer to problems identified by the client and are thus client specific and client delineated. Because these client health problems may take the form of decline of health and associated symptoms or the threat of loss of health, nursing care includes both treatment for existing health problems and preventive measures.

Societal Mandate for Nursing and the Discipline

As a profession, nursing is valued primarily for its deeds rather than its thoughts. Theorizing and knowledge development in nursing are supported because of the promise they offer for enlightened nursing practice (Donaldson & Crowley, 1978). The statements on standards for nursing practice (American Nurses' Association, 1973) have publicized nursing's commitment and intent to address societal health needs. Health promotion and illness prevention have been espoused as priorities for nursing practice (American Nurses' Association, 1980) and nursing research (National Center for Nursing Research, 1988). Fry (1981) studied the American standards and codes for practice and research and found that the concept of nursing encompasses technological skills and scientific knowledge and inquiry as well as humanistic caring and promotion of individual welfare/rights. Thus society has been promised scientific knowledge and science-based practice tempered by humanism and client participation in health decisions and outcomes (Gortner, 1990). Fulfillment of the promise is the primary source of societal credibility for the profession of nursing.

The discipline of nursing is, first and foremost, a practice discipline embodying prescriptive theories (Donaldson & Crowley, 1978). The discipline of nursing would wither if it were stripped of professional nursing practice or if the public's need for nursing services diminished. This central point often seems forgotten or misconstrued by those intent on developing the discipline and science of nursing. Although knowledge from the discipline may shape and expand practice, clinical service creates the demand for the development of the discipline, not vice versa. The discipline of nursing must, at a minimum, be a source of knowledge allowing the practice of nursing as explicated by its societal mandate.

Societal health needs are usually not expressed in terms of holism and self-actualization but, rather, as human misery. Human health-related misery may take many forms, including that resulting from medical therapies for the treatment and cure of disease or lifestyle changes requisite to the maintenance of health. Nurses must be prepared with effective strategies for the health problem that initiates the request for nursing service. The client's trust and willingness to engage in additional nursing care are determined by successful treatment of the presenting problem and its associated misery.

The current societal climate for health care is one of fiscal restraint and constraints concurrent with a demand for measurable client outcomes. This revolution in health care offers both a challenge and an opportunity for nursing. Jennings (1991) urges nurses to take a proactive role in patient outcomes research, especially since the existing research initiatives do not emphasize the nursing perspective of client outcomes. The opportunity for nursing is to advance theory for nursing practice (Jennings, 1991) and to interject a more holistic, autonomous perspective of the client (Gortner, 1990). The challenge to nursing is that failure to participate in health care reform may allow reshaping of nursing from sources beyond the profession.

Philosophical Bases of Nursing Science

SOURCES OF KNOWLEDGE
FOR THE NURSE PRAGMATIST

What is needed by the practicing professional nurse are well-tested theories and knowledge that allow conceptualization of the clinical problem and desired client outcomes, delineation of effective interventions, and measurement of client outcomes. Researchers and scholars who profess to build the discipline of nursing, including its science, should keep in mind that the centrality and value of this knowledge will be determined by the nurse pragmatist. The need to alleviate client health problems motivates the pragmatist, who uses any existing theory or knowledge relevant to their solution. From the "any which way you can" stance of the pragmatist, theory selection is eclectic, spanning distinct philosophies, paradigms, and disciplines. However, the pragmatist will employ knowledge from nursing and nursing science only if it has utility for achieving the desired clinical outcomes.

In the practice of nursing, nurses will, of necessity, draw information from many disciplines (Donaldson & Crowley, 1978). In formulating a plan of care, the nurse incorporates knowledge from the natural sciences and professional disciplines, such as education and medicine (Schultz & Meleis, 1988). Nursing interventions may involve physical manipulation of the client or the client's environment for which knowledge of the laws of physics is essential. Similarly, because nursing therapies must usually complement those of other health professionals, the nurse pragmatist must have knowledge from disciplines such as medicine and physical therapy. It is important to recognize that the nurse's entrée to the client is often through delegated clinical tasks; thus the trust of the client may hinge on the nurse's ability to effectively use received knowledge from medicine to intervene in a mode that is distinct from that of independent or autonomous nursing actions. The pragmatist would be concerned first with alleviation of the client's health problem and not with the classification of the nursing action. However, the pragmatist is not an intervention automaton; rather, the professional nurse pragmatist is tethered by the philosophy of nursing. Knowledge from the perspective of nursing is essential for the implementation of humanistic, holistic nursing care of the client. Thus the nurse pragmatist will rely on both the science and nonscience realms of the discipline of nursing (Donaldson & Crowley, 1978) in conceptualizing the client's health problem.

EMPIRICISM AND TRADITIONAL SCIENCE

By definition, the nurse pragmatist values most highly well-tested prescriptive theories. In selecting and planning interventions, the pragmatist will rely most heavily on knowledge generated within the paradigm of traditional science, primarily because scientific knowledge allows prediction of outcomes for observable or measurable real-world phenomena. Although explanation is not a priority for the nurse pragmatist, causal inference is essential (Gortner, 1990). Knowledge generated from rational philosophies and conceptual causal modeling will be sought and used to the extent that its empirical relevance has been demonstrated. Such knowledge is public in nature and is obtained through systematic inquiry that incorporates, as appropriate to the method (Leonard, 1989), the following: observation, logic, critical tests of theory and measures of validity/credibility, and reproducibility/ consistency.

This does not mean that the nurse pragmatist will subscribe strictly to logical positivism or the foundationalist philosophy of science in general. According to Schumacher and Gortner (1992), logical positivism, along with its claim to theory-neutral facts, has been discredited and should not be viewed, or represented, as contemporary philosophy of science. Logical positivism is the branch of foundationalism that seeks universal truths and eschews metaphysics. Contemporary philosophy of science, referred to as traditional science, seeks knowledge that is warranted by evidence and delineated by rational theory. Importantly, the warranting of knowledge in contemporary, traditional science is not constrained to a singular, uniform method requiring quantitative data. Rather, the traditional science paradigm for the realist includes qualitative and quantitative research (Gortner & Schultz, 1988). The phenomena of interest, not the paradigm, dictate the form of the data in contemporary traditional science. This is especially important to the pragmatist, who must address phenomena, such as coping processes, that are not observable or quantifiable.

As Schumacher and Gortner (1992) note, there is no historical or philosophical basis for equating traditional science with exclusively quantitative research; dating back to at least the 19th century, biologists used inductive reasoning and field notes within the paradigm of traditional science. Because the phenomena of interest to nursing include quantifiable and nonquantifiable, experiential phenomena, the discipline of nursing also embraces both quantitative and qualitative research. The naturalistic traditions of qualitative research are especially appealing to nursing because of the relevance of the phenomena of interest and because of the correspondence between the qualitative research philosophy and the values of nursing. According to Benner (1985), "Heideggerian phenomenology generates forms of explanation and prediction that offer understanding and choice, rather than manipulation and control" (p. 13).

The value of traditional science to the pragmatist is that it allows for generalization or application (Leonard, 1989) of findings beyond the sample of the study. As Schumacher and Gortner (1992) note, "If generalization were not allowed it would be difficult for clinicians to use the findings of research not conducted with their own patients" (p. 6). Scientific knowledge from the discipline of nursing will be especially useful to the nurse pragmatist because it has the advantage of being shaped by the nursing perspective, which values human autonomy and health.

Because the nurse pragmatist must deal with phenomena that are not always directly observable, the pragmatist will subscribe to the scientific realism branch of traditional science. Scientific realism, a branch of traditional science, allows for theoretical entities, causality, and explanation (Boyd, 1984). The antirealists, in contrast, carry forward the extreme position of denying the existence of entities that cannot be directly observed. Because nurses and nursing must deal with theoretical entities, such as human states and experiences, as well as real-world observable phenomena, the antirealist perspective is no better a fit with nursing than was that of logical positivism.

But as Schumacher and Gortner (1992) point out, the perspective of scientific realism is eminently appropriate for nursing. Scientific realists recognize the existence of theoretical entities or processes and use them to provide explanations for observable phenomena. The nurse pragmatist is less interested in the explanatory nature of theories within scientific realism than in the guidance for intervention that is derived from them; prediction per se does not offer these guidelines (Schumacher & Gortner, 1992).

CASUAL PARADIGMS

Schumacher and Gortner (1992) "do not argue for a given form of explanation; but simply claim that the idea of causation is necessary in nursing science because of its relevance for clinical practice" (p. 7). Acausal paradigms are embraced within the discipline of nursing because they offer the hope of a holistic view of human and humanness. However, if this knowledge is not communicated so as to have meaning for the pragmatist clinician, it is unlikely to be valued by the profession. This challenge of relevance for holistic approaches is exemplified in the following statement made by Morse, Bottorff, Neander, and Solberg (1991) to those who equate caring and nursing: "If caring is the 'central, dominant, and unifying feature of nursing,' then it must be relevant to practice and to the patient and not merely an internalized feeling on the part of the nurse" (p. 119). According to Hacking (1983), interventions should be aimed at causative states or processes. These are not required to be linear causal relationships. In the human sciences, causation may be complex and multidirectional (Schumacher & Gortner, 1992).

POSTSTRUCTURALISM AND NURSING SCIENCE

The preceding discussion addressed exclusively the structuralist perspective of science: the seeking of truth, order, and meaning for real-world phenomena. Poststructuralist scientists do not subscribe to these basic tenets of traditional science; rather, they view all phenomena as politics (Dreyfus & Rabinow, 1983). Knowledge is not factual but, rather, process and power for the poststructuralist scientist (Foucault,

1971/1977). This form of science also has a place in nursing to the extent that it provides knowledge to improve client health. Poststructuralist nurse scientists might reveal the bases for more enlightened societal/world health care policies. The use of knowledge as power could allow nurses to influence health care from a nursing perspective, that of enhancing autonomy of clients.

Pragmatism and a Unique Science of Nursing

The need for knowledge that is relevant to practice is shaping a unique science of nursing. Thorne (1991) argues that within the qualitative paradigm of research (including ethnography, phenomenology, and grounded theory) nurse scholars are shaping a research tradition that reflects the profession's unique biases as to applicability of the knowledge in the experiential domain of nursing practice. As Thorne (1991) notes, "The assumption that a research study will be incomplete without mention of some practical implications is evidence of nursing's departure from the projects of the more theoretically driven disciplines" (p. 185). This is also true for the quantitative research domain of the discipline of nursing. Knowledge gleaned from biological/physical methods used in nursing research builds primarily the discipline of nursing and may not "fit" the theoretical disciplines such as physiology, microbiology, and immunology (Donaldson & Crowley, 1978). Thus it appears that the nurse researchers remain pragmatists at heart and pragmatism rather than theoretical purity is shaping nursing's research traditions and the inherent nature of nursing science.

From the historicist's perspective, scientific progress is judged by the number of solved problems within a discipline (Laudan, 1977). In considering the discipline of nursing and nursing science, historicists Silva and Rothbart (1984) observe that "there will be less emphasis on truth and error as the criteria for assessing scientific progress and more emphasis on the actual solution to nursing care problems" (p. 12). They also see the clinician as being in an ideal position to assess whether, or to what degree, a nursing care problem has been solved. The nurse pragmatist will measure the utility of forms of nursing knowledge and various theories. This is understandable because, for a practice discipline, the significance of knowledge is derived from the meaning it has for human beings in terms of its effect on human suffering and individual capability (Baron, 1985).

A point of debate as to the role of the pragmatist in establishing utility of knowledge of the discipline of nursing is whether or not the client problems and nursing interventions are consistent with the prevailing philosophy of nursing. Throughout this chapter, this has been assumed. As noted before (Donaldson & Crowley, 1978), all the activities of practitioners are not necessarily nursing. Also, it is expected that the scope of the discipline of nursing will be broader than the current clinical practice of nursing; if clinical practice per se were to be the screen for defining the discipline, "professional nursing could be limited to functioning in the realm of disaster relief rather than serving as a force in the promotion of world health" (Donaldson & Crowley, 1978, p. 118). Thus scholars and researchers are free to expand the scope of nursing knowledge beyond the confines of current clinical practice, but the clinical usefulness of this knowledge will determine the success and scope of professional nursing. The challenge to theorists and researchers building the discipline and the science of nursing is to meet the needs of the nurse pragmatist so that both the discipline, which includes the science of nursing, and the profession thrive.

References

American Nurses' Association. (1973). *Standards of nursing practice*. Kansas City, MO: Author.

American Nurses' Association. (1980). *A social policy statement*. Kansas City, MO: Author.

Baron, R. (1985). An introduction to medical phenomenology: I can't hear you while I'm listening. *Annals of Internal Medicine, 163*, 606-611.

Benner, P. (1985). Quality of life: A phenomenological perspective on explanation, prediction, and understanding in nursing science. *Advances in Nursing Science, 8*(1), 1-14.

Boyd, R. N. (1984). The current status of scientific realism. In J. Leplin (Ed.), *Scientific realism* (pp. 41-58). Berkeley: University of California Press.

Dreyfus, H. L., & Rabinow, P. (1983). *Michel Foucault: Beyond structuralism and hermeneutics*. Chicago: University of Chicago Press.

Donaldson, S. K., & Crowley, D. M. (1978). The discipline of nursing. *Nursing Outlook, 26*(2), 113-120.

Foucault, M. (1977). Nietzsche, genealogy, and history. In D. F. Bouchard (Ed.). *Michel Foucault: Language, counter-memory, practice. Selected essays and interviews* (pp. 139-

164). New York: Cornell University Press. (Original work by Foucault published 1971)

Fry, S. (1981). Accountability in research: The relationship of scientific and humanistic values. *Advances in Nursing Science, 4*, 1-13.

Gortner, S. (1990). Nursing values and science: Toward a science philosophy. *Image: Journal of Nursing Scholarship, 22*(2), 101-108.

Gortner, S. R., & Schultz, P. R. (1988). Approaches to nursing science methods. *Image: Journal of Nursing Scholarship, 20*(1), 22-24.

Hacking, I. (1983). *Representing and intervening.* Cambridge: Cambridge University Press.

Jennings, B. M. (1991). Patient outcomes research: Seizing the opportunity. *Advances in Nursing Science, 14*(2), 59-72.

Laudan, L. (1977). *Progress and its problems: Towards a theory of scientific growth.* Berkeley: University of California Press.

Leonard, N. N. (1989). A Heideggerian phenomenologic perspective on the concept of person. *Advances in Nursing Science, 11*(4), 40-55.

Morse, J. M., Bottorff, J., Neander, W., & Solberg, S. (1991). Comparative analysis of conceptualizations and theories of caring. *Image: Journal of Nursing Scholarship, 23*(2), 119-126.

National Center for Nursing Research. (1988). *Nursing science: Serving health through research* [Program announcement]. Bethesda, MD: National Institutes of Health.

Schultz, P. R., & Meleis, A. I. (1988). Nursing epistemology: Traditions, insights, questions. *Image: Journal of Nursing Scholarship, 20*(4), 217-221.

Schumacher, K. L., & Gortner, S. R. (1992). (Mis)conceptions and reconceptions about traditional science. *Advances in Nursing Science, 14*(4), 1-11.

Silva, M. C., & Rothbart, D. (1984). An analysis of changing trends in philosophies of science on nursing theory development and testing. *Advances in Nursing Science, 6*(2), 1-13.

Thorne, S. E. (1991). Methodological orthodoxy in qualitative research: Analyses of the issues. *Qualitative Health Research, 1*(2), 178-199.

2

Contemporary Empiricism

SANDRA J. WEISS

Over the past decade, empiricism has incurred the wrath of some nurse scholars who believe that nursing science has been influenced negatively by empirical traditions. However, in the main, these opponents of empiricism remain fixated in the Kuhnian aftermath of the 1960s and 1970s when other disciplines were debating these issues. Their concerns focus primarily on the assumptions and methods of antiquated, positivistic notions that have limited influence in the contemporary empiricist paradigm. In reality, major changes have occurred in the empirical philosophy of science during the 1980s and 1990s. This chapter focuses on contemporary views of empiricism, as they are held by the majority of nurse scientists who employ empirical methods in their development of knowledge.

Assumptions Underlying Empiricism

Three major assumptions undergird an empirical philosophy of science. They reflect the understanding of the world and science that sets the stage for all tenets and methods of empiricism.

PREDICTABILITY VERSUS UNIVERSALITY

The first assumption is that some degree of predictability exists in the physical, psychological, and behavioral phenomena that make up the world as we know it. It is acknowledged that total predictability is neither realistic nor always desirable. There are many aspects of health and human responses that will never be fully understood. Since the original 17th-century view of empiricism, there has been recognition among empiricists that antecedent conditions cannot always predict the occurrence of some event. For example, the empirically based studies that generated "chaos theory" have created much intellectual excitement and a rethinking of traditional perspectives on explanation and prediction (Gleick, 1987).

No true scientist, or for that matter any intelligent human being, believes that the meaning of any phenomenon can ever be completely captured in all its complexities. Empiricism, like any approach to science, seeks only to further that understanding, to acquire a broader grasp of the dimensions that make up a phenomenon and the factors that may influence its perception, its occurrence, or its impact.

There is no belief by nurse empiricists in some totally uniform world that applies in every case. No common pattern is rigidly viewed as having relevance for every individual or situation. No universal laws governing all of health are believed to exist. Rather, there is the assumption that reasonable predictions are possible that can provide nurses with estimates of expected human responses under certain conditions of health and illness as well as how nursing care may serve to influence these responses in beneficial ways. The most typical empirical approach is to examine multiple environmental and person variables that may help to explain situational and individual differences in response patterns and to test theories suggesting multiple, interactive causal factors.

KNOWLEDGE TO IMPROVE NURSING PRACTICE

A second assumption is that the purpose of nursing science is to develop the basis for nursing care. Thus the societal commitment of all nurse scientists must be to generate knowledge that helps either to explain human responses associated with health and recovery from illness or to predict the effectiveness of various nursing interventions in bringing about these health-related goals. This commitment mandates greater explanatory power in whatever methods of science are employed. Explanation and prediction are seen as essential to defining the societal value of nursing research and maintaining the credibility of the nursing discipline. Since the 1950s, empiricists have recognized that the understanding of a phenomenon occurs not only through explanation but by a meticulous description of the phenomenon. Descriptive research from one study generates information for further exploration and testing. However, singular, descriptive studies cannot claim to provide credible knowledge that warrants being used as a guide for nursing practice.

ANALYSIS AND SYNTHESIS: UNDERSTANDING THE WHOLE

The last assumption is that human responses to health and illness can be identified, measured, and understood. This assumption places responsibility with the scientist to analyze *and* to synthesize phenomena so that their discrete properties, the relationships among these properties, and the meaning created by the synergism among all elements of the phenomenon can be clarified more fully. In other words, the meaning of the individual parts and of the whole are both seen as critical to knowledge development. In light of this assumption, it would be considered unacceptable to state that person and environment are inseparable for purposes of understanding. Indeed, they may be synergistic, creating a new meaning from the very fact of their transaction. However, they also constitute separate and distinct aspects of reality whose unique properties influence one another. Within empiricism, to eschew these unique contributions of important elements of the phenomenon would reflect fuzzy thinking, imprecision, and lack of attention to the nuances constituting full knowledge of the phenomenon.

This analytic component of empiricism has been demeaned by some nurse philosophers as reducing the larger phenomenon to parts that by themselves cannot be understood as representing the phenomenon as a whole. Nurse scientists who are true to empiricism would agree completely with this concern. Within the empirical paradigm, knowledge development is considered a long-term trajectory that involves breaking down a phenomenon to carefully examine its properties, testing hypotheses gleaned from this analysis, reassessing the properties in light of new knowledge, testing new hypotheses, studying relationships in light of the whole, and so forth and so on. Researchers who conduct one study involving one part of a phenomenon in isolation and who never continue the entire trajectory so as to synthesize various aspects of the whole are not upholding the values of empiricism. The paradigm should not be judged by evaluation of those who are not true empiricists but have only employed certain of its methods inappropriately.

Major Tenets of Empiricism

Diversification rather than unification is the distinctive feature of contemporary empiricism. Consequently, multiple perspectives exist as to how one should conceptualize the empirical philosophy of science. However, there are two major tenets that serve as the foundation for all empirical thought: deductive reasoning and substantiation of theoretical claims.

DEDUCTIVE REASONING

The "pure" empiricists of the 17th century believed that all hypotheses must stem from experience. Inductive hunches were generated from sensory data; that is, what could be seen, heard, touched. The logical positivists of the early 1930s continued with this approach, often developing their hypotheses from the data of one experiment. Then came the logical empiricists who declaimed being called positivists specifically because of the positivists' reliance on inductive reasoning. Logical empiricists proposed instead a "hypothetico-deductive" approach that was "theory driven." Karl Popper (1962) was a major force behind this change. He proposed that inductive inference was inadequate to support claims of knowledge and instead substituted a process of deduction whereby one begins with a hypothesis or, better yet, alternative hypotheses that reflect different theories regarding a particular phenomenon.

The requirements of a hypothetico-deductive approach are that empirical data (evidence from particular events or experiences) are a logical consequence of, or correspond to, a specific theory and its related hypotheses. Deductivism prescribes that a theory that cannot be falsified in test after test of its hypotheses should be regarded as having the greatest likelihood of being accurate or valid knowledge. The approach of deductivism rests with falsifying or refuting alternative theories rather than trying to achieve confirmation or support for a particular theory from one or two tests. A theory must be able to withstand repeated tests without being refuted for it to be taken seriously.

Objectivity

As Gortner (1987) points out, this approach helps to guard against biases in seeking support for some "favored hunch." Empiricism requires that all scientific reasoning must be as free of bias as is humanly possible. This expectation in no way represents some ignorant belief that total objectivity can ever occur. Nurse empiricists acknowledge that the experiential and conceptual background of the scientist as well as her or his unique constellation of personality traits may influence the values brought to the scientific process. These factors can affect not only the hunches developed but the methods to test them and the interpretation of the findings. To some extent, the influence of these factors is inevitable because the researcher brings to any study of a phenomenon a history of prior experience with it. The empiricist is expected to make the commitment to extract oneself, as much as possible, from preconceptions that would prejudge outcomes of research to the exclusion of other possibilities. This commitment has existed from the time of Francis Bacon (1621/1889).

Deductive reasoning facilitates objectivity by encouraging examination of a phenomenon in light of findings from previous research, conceptualizations contributed by other scholars, and testing of more than one prediction. Objectivity is thus enhanced while recognizing that biases can never be fully precluded.

Theoretical Models

Theoretical models are the core of deductive reasoning. They are considered useful abstract schemes for classifying many specific samplings of common situations and relating events or experiences in a way that suggests more general application. A theoretical model is a system of inference with specific concepts that reflect the ideas or elements essential to the understanding of a phenomenon and hypotheses clarifying the relationships among these concepts. A theory is not one simple hypothesis but synthesizes a body of hypotheses or connected set of propositions. Its purposes are to provide as complete a picture of the phenomenon as possible and to serve as the basis for prediction and explanation of the phenomenon. The additional value of theoretical models is their ability to simplify and organize diverse and complex bodies of information.

The dangers of models include the potential for grossly oversimplifying reality and relationships and the potential for missing important new knowledge because it does not fit within the model's existing definition of the phenomenon. This latter danger was the concern of the logical positivists, who argued that a theoretical model distorts the unique character of the individual events or experience that the scientist is trying to explain. If these pitfalls are to be avoided, nurse scientists must always take them seriously and keep their likelihood in the forefront of consciousness. As Wilson-Barnett (1991) has pointed out, "Failure to be open-minded . . . and exploit unexpected results would be the mark of an inept researcher in whatever camp (s)he was placed" (p. 84). Theories are merely intellectual constructions with uncertain links; they must, therefore, be critically examined and their propositions tested over and over again.

Theoretical models can be of two types: deterministic and probabilistic (Giere, 1984). Deterministic models propose that an initial set of conditions at one point in time completely determines the state of a phenomenon at all other times. This view of reality would assume that all human responses or health states are precisely and completely determined by preceding events or factors in an individual's or family's life. Such a model leaves no room for the modifying or interactive effects of the environment or for the individual's ability to actively modify the effects of some "givens" at birth. The most deterministic of models assume that the universe is orderly, with every outcome having a cause that is sole and sufficient. An example of a hypothesis based on a deterministic model is the following: For patients with a specific disease, one type of nursing intervention would lead to recovery whereas another would inhibit recovery. An even more specific example is the hypothesis that, given a genetic vulnerability to eating disorders, an unsupportive family environment makes the crucial difference in development of anorexia. Deterministic models are tied to the belief in universal laws governing all situations at all times. This belief system was dominant in the 18th and 19th centuries but has little hold on empiricism today. As science has matured, the implausibility of such a view in our complex world has been recognized.

Probabilistic (or stochastic) models propose that a set of initial conditions or factors determine only the probability of various possible responses or outcomes at later times. This approach reflects the relative frequency or degree of likelihood of a certain response based on preceding conditions or events. Probabilistic models never assume that any theory will be true in all cases as some universal rule. An example of a hypothesis based on a probabilistic model is that for patients with a specific disease, some nursing interventions have a higher probability than others of influencing patient recovery. A probabilistic hypothesis regarding eating disorders looks very different from the one described earlier. For example, given a genetic vulnerability to eating disorders, an unsupportive family environment may influence the probability of developing the disorder, but the probability will be different for different people based on certain modifying factors, such as personality, other sources of social support, and degree of life stress.

Probabilistic models are the obvious choice of nurse empiricists today. The challenge is to develop coherent theories that can be useful in *guiding* nursing practice, not to determine some standardized protocol to be applied for every patient with certain health problems or response patterns.

SUBSTANTIATION OF THEORETICAL CLAIMS

The second major tenet within an empirical philosophy of science is substantiation. No theoretical claim should ever be given "truth" status. All claims regarding a phenomenon are considered merely plausible. Any theory must be subjected to extensive testing to establish the "truth" of its claims. This process involves some logical formulation of the specific operations to be performed to test the theory and how these operations will make the abstract ideas or hypotheses observable.

Making Hypotheses Observable

Observations are a fundamental cornerstone of substantiation and have held a place of value within the empirical tradition from its origins in the late 17th century to the present. Hypotheses cannot be tested unless they can be translated into concrete behaviors, thoughts, or feelings that can be measured, that is, observed in some form other than in the language or thoughts of the scientist. Observation implicates the senses, so that what can be perceived through experience is the source of all knowledge. Experience is viewed as providing evidence of what is "real" in the world. Early empiricists believed that no preconceptions of the world existed until our experience gave us data from which to form abstract ideas and understand the world. This original phenomenal view of knowledge (i.e., knowing through the senses rather than through thought or intuition) was modified substantially in Locke's (1924) theory of knowledge. He proposed that people bring a unique contribution to this sensory input by virtue of their ability to reflect on sensory experience. Thus not everything was strictly phenomenal but involved interpretation by the individual. Locke's theory was the first empirical recognition of the importance of subjective experience resulting from the interaction between the properties inherent in the object or event being experienced and the unique perceptions of the individual who was experiencing it. In this way, the human mind makes "a cherry" of a small, red, smooth, sweet object by unifying sensations of sight, taste, and touch and giving it an abstract label through an interpretation of the whole. Clearly, even in the early stages of empiricism, the interaction between person and environment carried weight. Whereas logical positivists reverted to a strict focus on phenomenalism (sense data as the sole source of knowledge—pure facts), the logical empiricists of later years saw the need to reconnect experience with human interpretation. Abstract ideas and sensory data were viewed as interdependent by the logical empiricists (Hempel, 1965). Conceptualization helped to organize experience to better understand the sensory data, and the observable data were viewed as essential to the meaning of any conceptualization.

For all empiricists, verbal conceptualization has been considered problematic because various idiomatic expressions surrounding words used by scientists have led to ambiguity and unreliable understanding of meanings being shared. This "ontological confusion" (Turner, 1965) was the source of emphasis on operational definitions of terms and quantification (i.e., mathematical language) that had no conceptual reference that could be misinterpreted and extended beyond the exact measurement index used in a particular situation or experience.

The concept of "observation" has been distorted by many skeptics of the empirical approach who define it as something "outside" the human being, as if, somehow, experience does not include feelings, opinions, or attitudes. No contemporary nurse empiricist would accept such a definition. As Gortner (1990) notes, "To be observable means that measurement is possible" (p. 104). Observation implies the ability to define and capture an aspect of experience through valid and reliable instrumentation. Emotions (e.g., anxiety) and thoughts (e.g., identification of stressors) are central to experience and represent a major focus of empirical work in nursing as do physiologic responses (e.g., heart rate) and behavior (e.g., exercise regimes or parenting practices). All of these important dimensions of human response can be measured to yield empirical data, and as such they represent "observations" in the empirical sense.

Operations to Test the Theory

The "experiment" has traditionally been the means through which empiricists tested assertions regarding knowledge. The experimental approach originated with Mill (1884) and his followers. They pushed for more than observing, classifying, and counting phenomena—that is, meticulous description of the experience. Mill identified the need for repeated trials to isolate and verify factors that seemed to bring about a particular outcome and then to modify or add some other factor and observe its effect. He proposed that if two factors varied together in a consistent and persistent fashion the concomitant variation represented either a direct causal relationship or both factors were being similarly influenced by some other causal factor. The logical positivists of the early 20th century built on this work by insisting that all claims of knowledge be verified through experimental confirmation. Although they attempted to show support for an idea through an experiment, they often accepted the "truth" of the idea based on evidence from one experiment. This resulted in Popper's (1961) proposal that claims regarding knowledge must not simply be verified but be subjected to falsification. This stance saw the experiment as a means to hold or reject a theory based on testing alternative hypotheses. Popper (1979) described "the growth of our knowledge [as] . . . a competitive struggle which eliminates those hypotheses which are unfit" (p. 261). The hypotheses to be tested were stated to contradict what was expected, and then attempts were made to falsify them. If a particular set of hypotheses failed to be falsified after repeated trials under different conditions, then and only then could a theory be considered a likely candidate for substantiation.

Beyond the need to tighten up standards for substantiation of claims, logical empiricists recognized that some theories could never be verified by some finite set of observations but still could be essential to the chain of scientific inference. For instance, speculation regarding the existence of genes had no direct evidence to confirm it for years. As long as such a theory could not be falsified it should remain plausible.

The accepted view of an experiment has traditionally included some form of controlled comparison between two groups of subjects, one of which was exposed to some manipulation of an independent or explanatory variable while the other did not experience the manipulation. Different outcomes with regard to some dependent variable of theoretical interest were then compared. The controlled aspect of the comparison involved minimizing the effects of extraneous variables that could modify the outcomes for one or both groups. The conditions of the experiment were thus carefully delineated and the effects of certain variables precluded by strict sampling procedures to randomize, or to exclude the possibility of certain variables confounding the procedures.

These experimental principles are still applied in empirical studies of phenomena that can be realistically researched in controlled environments and that are being examined within the context of a highly parsimonious theoretical model. However, most contemporary theoretical models are more complex than simple; they recognize the plurality of causation and the multiplicity of potential modifying or confounding variables. It has been widely understood for years that definitive experiments are impossible, that their goal is merely better understanding, not full prediction or control (Cronbach & Snow, 1977). All sources of error need not be eliminated entirely to discover some generalizable patterns that can provide useful knowledge (Serlin, 1987). In today's complex scientific world, it is recognized that explanation is not precise in the sense it was expected to be half a century ago.

Regardless of these constraints, some coherent understanding of a phenomenon is very possible. Because nursing science addresses human responses within highly complex social, biological, and psychological environments, the pragmatic difficulties in creating a controlled situation or eliminating sources of error are myriad. Use of statistical procedures to examine the influence of, or potential variance contributed by, certain modifying factors is often viewed as far more valuable (and more feasible) than trying to eliminate the influence of the factor. By eliminating it, its causal, interactive, or modifying effects are never understood. Thus multivariate statistics have increased in their application along with the need for much larger samples to provide the power necessary for testing the effects of multiple variables. Causal modeling is an example of a contemporary approach to explanation. Data are examined for how they fit with different conceptual models using this multivariate approach. Different explanatory variables can be built into the statistical modeling to evaluate the degree of variance they contribute (as independent, interactive, or modifying influences) to selected outcomes.

This is not to say that nurse empiricists do not use the highly controlled comparison of some experimental manipulation as an important way to test hypotheses and build explanatory models to guide practice. Rather, there are many methods employed within contemporary empiricism that are unique to the complexity of the phenomenon and the stage of knowledge development for the particular phenomenon.

Procedures used within contemporary empiricism also attend to the careful delineation of the context or conditions under which evaluation has occurred. There is no attempt to achieve complete "control" over the conditions, a requisite put forward by the logical empiricists of the mid 20th century. Instead, factors within the context of the phenomenon that are suspected of having some influence are identified, held constant if possible, or, more frequently, included in the analysis to determine their role in contributing to the phenomenon. One does not need to include all possible variables, only those that could play a role in the phenomenon or theory being tested (Lehrer, Serlin, & Amundson, 1990).

Context is of central consideration in the substantiation of any theoretical claims. At the very minimum, empiricism necessitates a full description of the conditions under which the phenomenon occurs. For the majority of nurse empiricists, this contextual description also includes qualitative data from open-ended questions or interviews to augment the understanding of the numerical data acquired. As the testing of a theory progresses, the details of the context become further refined, individual differences are clarified that may influence the meaning of the phenomenon, and other variables that may need incorporation are added to the model. Identification of what constitutes the context versus key explanatory variables is rethought and reshaped over successive phases of testing. This careful delineation of context has a twofold purpose. First, it is necessary so as to assure that interpretations of the generalizability of the experiment's findings do not go beyond the bounds of "truth." The actual conditions determine the applicability of any assertions across population and situation. Second, in the course of repeated trials to further test the hypothesis, it is essential that there is clarity regarding the exact conditions under which the phenomenon was studied. Otherwise, claims of reproducibility cannot be made or subtle changes in conditions that affect the findings cannot be understood.

In sum, experimental operations provide the basis for determining whether theoretical claims are warranted. They tell us when modifications are called for in hypotheses, how we should confine the range of a theory's application, or that testing of a proposed hypothesis should be continued because it holds promise as a plausible explanation in our understanding of the health phenomenon being studied.

The Significance of Empiricism for Nursing

It would be naive to view any one paradigm as the only true scientific paradigm, but, as Norbeck (1987) has stated, "the empiricist perspective . . . should be a dominant perspective in nursing research because many of the questions that we need to study are consistent with this view" (p. 29).

Nursing research must be meaningful in terms of its contribution to improved health or more effective nursing practice. In other words, our scientific inquiry must produce tangible, concrete knowledge that promotes health, prevents illness, or increases the potential for recovery from illness. If not, nursing science does not warrant any commitment of societal resources to it, and, as nurse scientists, we are not meeting our obligations to society. Mere understanding is not an adequate rationale for nursing research.

Contemporary empiricism provides a systematic structure for both scientific reasoning and substantiation of claims regarding health-related responses and nursing care. This structure assists in reducing bias and error and developing explanatory models to guide effective nursing practice. As Gortner (1990) points out, the absence of these factors in science could have "serious implications for the human sciences in general and the health sciences in particular. There is loss of generalizability, loss of correspondence with extant theory, and diminished power to make . . . inferences that can extend research and therapy" (p. 103).

Empiricism has served the health sciences well in these important areas of knowledge development. As a philosophy of science, it warrants major emphasis in nursing if we are to achieve full recognition as a health science discipline and maximize our contributions to society.

References

Bacon, F. (1889). *Novum organum*. Oxford: Oxford University Press. (Original work published 1621)

Cronbach, L., & Snow, R. (1977). *Aptitudes and instructional methods*. New York: Irvington.

Giere, R. (1984). *Understanding scientific reasoning*. New York: Holt, Rinehart & Winston.

Gleick, J. (1987). *Chaos: Making a new science*. New York: Viking.

Gortner, S. (1987). *Nursing science methods: A reader*. San Francisco: University of California Press.

Gortner, S. (1990). Nursing values and science: Toward a science philosophy. *Image: Journal of Nursing Scholarship, 22*(2), 101-105.

Hempel, C. (1965). *Aspects of scientific explanation and other essays in the philosophy of science*. New York: Free Press.

Lehrer, R., Serlin, R., & Amundson, R. (1990). Knowledge or certainty? *Educational Researcher, 19*(6), 16-19.

Locke, J. (1924). *An essay concerning human understanding*. Oxford: Clarendon.

Mill, J. (1884). *A system of logic*. London: Longmans.

Norbeck, J. (1987). In defense of empiricism. *Image: Journal of Nursing Scholarship, 19*(1), 28-30.

Popper, K. (1961). *The logic of scientific discovery*. New York: John Wiley.

Popper, K. (1962). *Conjectures and refutations.* New York: Harper.

Popper, K. (1979). *Objective knowledge: An evolutionary approach.* Oxford: Clarendon.

Serlin, R. (1987). Hypothesis testing, theory building, and the philosophy of science. *Journal of Counseling Psychology, 34,* 365-371.

Turner, M. (1965). *Philosophy and the science of behavior.* New York: Appleton-Century-Crofts.

Wilson-Barnett, J. (1991). The experiment: Is it worthwhile? *International Journal of Nursing Studies, 28*(1), 77-87.

3

Pragmatism

The Problem With the Bottom Line

CHRISTINE E. KASPER

This chapter reviews the origins and structure of historical philosophic pragmatic thought and illustrates how professional nursing hinders its ability to attain its broad biopsychosocial patient care goals by ascribing to "pragmatism."

Philosophic Pragmatism

Traditional academic philosophy, especially that of logical positivism and operationism, has sought to clarify the meaning of statements. These traditions seek not only to clarify the meaning and truth of a statement but also the process or method used to reach this goal. These methods are also known as semantic empiricism. Pragmatism differs from these philosophic views in that it is primarily a method of evaluating philosophy by investigating problems and clarifying communication. It does not seek to clarify the meaning and truth of statements, nor does it find ultimate answers or great truths. Pragmatism focuses on the "outcome variable." Stated in another way, if the statement in question were true, what difference would it make to us (Kaplan, 1967)? Pragmatism is a part of a greater pursuit of inquiry and truth. In this role, pragmatism has helped shape modern philosophy as a method of investigating problems and clarifying communication versus a fixed system of ultimate answers and great truths.

Using the pragmatic method, the test of a statement's meaningfulness is whether or not it ultimately makes a difference or matters to us. Consequently, the statement's meaning is solely defined by the difference that it makes in knowledge, development of ideas, and the conduct of life.

The pragmatic method differs from traditional epistemic empiricism in that it focuses on the future and outcomes and not on the origins of the statement (Kaplan, 1967). The goals of this method are to provide undisputed definitional clarity of statements and to judge the value of an idea by its practical consequences.

For the pragmatist, the capacity to know "truth" is inseparable from purpose and action. To accomplish a purpose, one must proceed to act in accordance with the meaning. Meaning and purpose are closely linked if not synonymous. Peirce (1961) stated that every meaningful statement may determine the correlation between desire and action. Operationally speaking, each statement is linked to a specific action that produces a defined outcome.

A nursing example of this approach, for example, is similar to the treatment of a patient based on tightly defined actions to produce a specific outcome criteria. Today, this method of health care has been institutionalized as DRGs (diagnostic related groups), critical pathways, and protocols (Bender, 1990; Hollander, Smith, & Barron, 1992; Omachonu & Nanda, 1989) where nursing care is tightly linked to time-based schedules of treatment and similarly timed patient outcomes. Therefore, a statement can be understood only in the context of the action that we would take in all similar circumstances. There is no meaning other than the plan of action (Kaplan, 1967); therefore, knowledge is contextual and outcome driven.

Historical Origins of Pragmatic Thought

Historically, pragmatism became the most important and influential philosophy in the United States during the early 20th century. Pragmatism is unique as an energetically evolved philosophical movement and, in contrast to other branches of philosophical thought, is perhaps best understood as an evolving movement rather than a singular doctrine (Prado, 1987).

As a movement, pragmatism sought to critically reject traditional academic philosophies and focus on positive aims and outcomes. Due to this unusual philosophical stance, the pragmatic movement distinguished itself as a unique and major contribution to philosophy in general. Many European philosophers such as Henri Bergson, Giovanni Vailati, Hans Hahn, Georg Simel, Wilhelm Ostwald, and Edmund Husserl were heavily influenced by the early pragmatists (Goetz, 1990).

Pragmatism as a method of philosophizing was first developed by Charles Peirce in the 1870s (Rorty, 1962, 1966, 1971), redefined by William James in 1898 as a theory of truth (Rorty, 1962; Wiener, 1973), and widely promoted by F.C.S. Schiller and John Dewey. The development of pragmatic thought appears to have occurred within the context of the "Metaphysical Club," which was organized by Peirce, James, and others in Cambridge, Massachusetts during the 1870s (Rorty, 1971; Wiener, 1973). It is interesting to note that even though this philosophic method was developed within the close working relationships of this "Club," its participants later expressed widely divergent interpretations of their individual understanding of the "pragmatic" method.

Owing to its confused historical origins, the precise philosophical definition and interpretation of pragmatism remain obscure. It is therefore simpler to regard pragmatic doctrine as an associated group of ideas developed over time that may differ, depending on whether Peirce's, James's, or Dewey's writing is used. It appears to be the consensus of modern philosophers that the development of a central, definitive statement of the tenants of pragmatism is highly unlikely to occur (Gallie, 1952; Rorty, 1962; Wiener, 1973). It is also interesting to note that since 1878 when Peirce set forth his ideas in the paper "How to Make Our Ideas Clear" the pragmatists have experienced great difficulties in making their philosophy succinct and understandable (Buchler, 1955).

Key Concepts of Pragmatic Science

The central themes of pragmatic science center around two main issues: clarity of ideas and the meaning, truth, and value of ideas as judged by their practical consequences. These two lines of thought are complementary and do not necessarily need to operate together.

Clarity of ideas, or conceptual clarity, is necessary to provide the clear and unambiguous use of words. In many ways, this is similar to that of a well-written research hypothesis. Using the same analogy, a description of specific aims of any research proposal gives the broad background and assumptions; it is the hypotheses that succinctly and precisely define the question. If a clear hypothesis cannot be stated, then that question cannot be successfully investigated.

For any concept, method, or idea to be of worth there must always be practical consequences. All meanings, truths, and value of ideas are judged by whether they are useful—do they have a quantifiable "bottom line"? If a concept or idea cannot be clearly defined and cannot provide evidence of concrete useful outcomes, then that issue is not deemed to be of worth. Unfortunately at this time, much of nursing science and practice cannot be clearly defined or provide evidence of useful outcomes.

Key Concepts Related to
Individual Authors and Their Relationships

The evolution and core of the pragmatic school of thought is centered on the works of Pierce, James, and Dewey. Since the origination of this philosophic method, little novel or innovative work has been added to these core works.

The general approach described by Peirce (1961) for the clarification of statements is not unlike the current use of the concepts and methods of the "scientific method" or "nursing process." Each assumption, assertion, or action is defined within the context of a closely delineated set of assumptions for a given case (Hartshorne, Weiss, & Burks, 1931-1958; Kaplan, 1967; Peirce, 1961). In reality, the most difficult part of Peirce's methods is the ability to obtain absolute clarity of definition, as all meanings are subject to the context in which they are used and all contexts vary, depending on the societal and cultural values used for each assumption.

The pragmatic method, according to Peirce, is best defined as a way of supporting clarity of speech and concepts and was intended to be applied to discussions of intellectual problems. By maintaining clarity of speech through the use of the pragmatic method, the path to the outcome would become self-evident. Peirce was known to state that pragmatism was not a philosophy or a theory of truth but "a technique to help us find solutions to problems of a philosophical or scientific nature" (quoted in Wiener, 1973, p. 433).

For example, Peirce stated in his 1878 paper "How to Make Our Ideas Clear," "Consider what effects, that might conceivably have practical bearings, we conceive the object of our conception to have. Then our conception of these effects is the whole of our conception of the objects." Later, he clarified this by stating, "In order to ascertain the meaning of an intellectual conception one should consider what practical consequences might conceivably result by necessity from the truth of that conception; and the sum of these consequences will constitute the entire meaning of the conception" (quoted in Wiener, 1973, p. 432). In short, Peirce defined his pragmatism as a method of procedures for promoting linguistic and conceptual clarity, where the emphasis is on the method and process of clarifying the meaning of words, ideas, and concepts and the aim is to facilitate communication. To quote one of Peirce's more brief and concise statements, "Pragmatism solves no real problem. It only shows that supposed problems are not real problems" (quoted in Wiener, 1973, p. 432).

The second part of Peirce's methods of clarification of statements deals with the interpretation of "signs." These signs are held to be ideas, concepts, and language. The method provides for a systematic approach to "translating" a word or statement into other words or statements that are concise, clear, and have an undisputed meaning. Terms that need to be clarified are always stated in the context of a given situation that operationally defines the terms and produces a specific result. All signs are essentially given in terms of this operational definition and are called "prescription" or "precept" (Buchler, 1955). They are always to be considered in the context of the effect that a given derived conclusion has on "practical" or "sensible" effects. Concepts and signs must always have practical consequences.

In contrast to Peirce, William James viewed pragmatism as a concrete level of experience infused with a strong moralistic undertone. In his famous work, *Pragmatism,* James (1907) states, "The whole function of philosophy ought to be to find out what definite difference it will make to you and me, at definite instants of our life, if this world-formula or that world-formula be the true one" (quoted in Wiener, 1973, p. 433). James judges meaning, truth, and value of ideas by whether or not they have definite practical consequences in terms of usefulness. James used an early 20th-century version of the term " bottom line" to describe an idea's worth as its "cash value" (Wiener, 1973).

For James, truth was the ability to think clearly and with a purpose that had a positive social value. If ideas were clearly linked to behavior, then society would benefit from labor saving, social well-being, and simplicity in all things. In comparison to Peirce, these ideas were focused on the immediate experience to promote utility of purpose (Rorty, 1962; Wiener, 1973).

John Dewey viewed James as a humanist and Peirce as a logician. In his paper, "The Development of American Pragmatism," Dewey (1931) took the concepts and ideas of Peirce and James and completely reformulated pragmatism into what he named "instrumentalism" (see also Wiener, 1973). Instrumentalism was defined as "a theory of the general forms of conception and reasoning" and combined both the theory of logic and a prescriptive outline of ethical analysis and criticism. Dewey felt that this philosophy would combine the dualisms of the separation of science and morals and knowledge and morals. It focused on the processes of thought, what controlled these processes, and how these thoughts would then control future outcomes.

Recent views of pragmatism have stressed what is known as "conceptual pragmatism," that is, the incorporation of the role that individual and social values play on our interpretation of experience. This twist on conventional pragmatism was first described by C. I. Lewis in 1920. Lewis (1929) clearly exposes one of the greatest weaknesses of pragmatic thought with his work: Specifically, the utility of our actions and processes of thought are largely determined by the social or individual value system used to infer meaning. According to Lewis,

The interpretation of experience must always be in terms of categories . . . and concepts which the mind itself determines. There may be alternative conceptual systems giving rise to alternative descriptions of experience, which are equally objective and equally valid. When this is so, choice will be determined, consciously or unconsciously, on pragmatic ground. (p. 375)

Therefore, to fully use pragmatism as a method of attributing meaning to communication or to promote conceptual clarity to intellectual problems, one must always be aware of the value system that one is using.

Operationalism

Operationalism is similar to pragmatism in that it is also a form of semantic empiricism. Used in the form of "operational definitions," operationalism became very popular with the behavioral sciences. In essence, every definition or description was placed in the context of use. The context of use serves as a clarification of the definition used, and meaning is derived from the situation of use (Kaplan, 1967).

In the process of scientific research, each measurement or use of a technical instrument can only be interpreted in terms of the set of operations used to carry out the measurement. If, for example, the room temperature changes or the location of the thermometer is different, one could not generalize from one experiment to another. Unfortunately, operational approaches have not developed methods to determine which variables are important and which are not. The conduct of data collection during "real" research requires one to only be aware of the status of intervening variables when one is unable to control them all. However, the use of operational definitions does permit a cautious comparison between scientific studies to derive meaning, and it is this comparison that is important as it constitutes scientific knowledge.

Assumptions

The most important driving assumption of pragmatism is that all knowledge depends on the value systems used to interpret the data. The value systems used during interpretation of data are important not only because they influence the way in which any data are analyzed but because the very control of the values of that belief system contains great political power to interpret data and ascribe significance and worth according to one's own values. Control can and often does lead to bias. The risks of unethical application and manipulation of this method are great.

In general, the use of pragmatic methods and operationalism permit us to clarify the meaning of complex questions, thoughts, and definitions and permits the interpretation of data within a set of known circumstances. The ultimate utility of these endeavors must always be interpreted with a clear and conscious knowledge of the social, scientific, and personal value systems that are used to perform the interpretation. Given the knowledge that all depends on the value systems used to interpret an idea or circumstance, it becomes very clear that the nature of reality is variable or "plastic." If the nature of reality is plastic and dependent on the value system used to interpret data, then considerable control can be exercised socially and politically in a given population by declaring an action or judgment useful and practical. The one who controls the value system will control the outcome of any plan of action.

QUANTITATIVE DRIVES OUT THE NONQUANTITATIVE OR THE "BOTTOM LINE"

People operate with distinct covert philosophies, and, in trying to understand how they differ, it is very tempting to take a bottom-line approach. But there are inherent drawbacks in taking that kind of approach, most particularly the tendency for the quantitative to drive out the nonquantitative. Nonquantitative variables are found in the humanities as well as in social and cultural value systems. When these variables are removed from the decision-making process in deference to a quantitative bottom-line approach, society, humanity, and the future are often irreparably harmed and one's quality of life is somehow diminished.

The concept of the "bottom line" is used to state that which is the most basic or core unit of understanding a situation or piece of information. We often hear statements such as "X, Y, and Z are wonderful, but the bottom line is that we need to adhere to this month's budget." Again, the question of values, culture, and individual interpretation influence what the bottom line is stated to be. It may not be the same for all groups involved in the same set of circumstances. Often, the only value considered is that of the acquisition of personal power and control.

A seductive use of this approach to decision making involves the use of quantitative data to influence or support a certain point of view. A mathematical number appears to be definite, discrete, and easily understood. Numbers are used to convey certainty and clarity to variables, and society tends to view quantitative data without undue suspicion. Somehow, there is psychological comfort in the ability to distill the essence of any question to a concrete, quantifiable number. Here, the unseen land mines of interpretation exist whenever the "hidden agenda," or operational definition, is not made explicitly clear. All too often, we are unable to clarify our methods of bestowing pragmatic meaning because our individual and societal prejudices are too hidden or unconscious to be publicly declared.

If You Can't Quantify It, It Doesn't Exist

It is a pervasive belief that if you cannot quantify a phenomenon, it does not exist in reality. This belief system is another that contributes to the misuse and abuse of the bottom-line mentality. Ignoring phenomena that have been observed or hypothesized solely by virtue of an inability to quantify them reflects another method of controlling which meanings and variables participate in defining the bottom line. Unfortunately, the prestige of "hard" quantifiable science is greatly valued in our culture.

An alternate view of this situation may be demonstrated using the recent growth and development of the science and theory of chaos. Complex systems, especially those of human physiology, have traditionally been viewed as not quantifiable. Many of these phenomena, such as cardiac arrhythmias, have been described as random, unstable, and unpredictable. Methods to quantify arrhythmias did not exist. Recently, the mathematical discipline of nonlinear dynamics or the theory of chaos has developed methods to describe and quantify these and similar phenomena.

Besides cardiac arrhythmias, phenomena that have been shown to be chaotic are transition to turbulence in fluids, mechanical vibrations, the rise and fall of epidemics, and leaking faucets (Garfinkel, Spano, Ditto, & Weiss, 1992). Chaos is a mathematical concept that is best defined as deterministic randomness. It is deterministic as it arises from internal causes and not from external sources, and it has the attribute of randomness as it is irregular and demonstrates unpredictable behavior (Pool, 1989). The major challenge that existed in defining these phenomena was developing a model of the system that was sufficiently detailed to identify the key parameters. Once these key parameters were identified, the ability to alter the system existed. A limiting factor in this example is the ability to use a system where a theoretical model is known and does not display irreversible parametric changes.

Chaos theory has begun quantifying and describing previously qualitative phenomena in such diverse fields as atmospheric behavior in meteorology, business cycles in economics, brain wave patterns in physiology, war behavior in international politics, star pulsations in astronomy, and snarled traffic patterns in transportation. So, in some ways it may be regarded as a pragmatic theory. These phenomena always existed; however, a method to measure them did not. It is possible that the observable but not yet quantifiable phenomenon of nursing may also be eventually quantified.

A bottom-line approach that depends on quantitative data is often used to "rationally" remove or destroy those things that are largely qualitative. For example, today many large state universities are seriously underfunded due to the depressed national and local economies. These administrative units seek to streamline their methods of delivering education and conducting research by decreasing personnel and programs. Their bottom line is to adhere to a limited budget.

The process of downsizing a major university involves many administrative actions and choices that are driven by the value systems of the administrators in charge. For example, which departments and disciplines are valued and which are not? What is the specific value system employed? History has repeatedly demonstrated that when budget cuts are needed within the context of a university medical center, it is the nursing staff, faculty, and students that are expendable. The hidden value system used in this instance is that (a) the cash flow produced by physicians is more valuable than a high level of quality of care, (b) nurses do not directly generate cash flow and thereby do not control the situation, and (c) schools of nursing tend not to generate large financial endowments and are expendable, and so forth and so on. Social need, care of the indigent, or contribution to quality of life and the alleviation of suffering are never taken into consideration. When questioned, the administrators point to the quantifiable budget as the basis of their actions. They plead that their actions are not constrained by ethics or moral choices as their decisions are based solely on a quantifiable variable that must be adhered to.

Control Can Lead to Bias

Given that our society bestows great prestige on quantitative science, every effort is made to pursue quantifiable research topics. Unfortunately, quantitative science is not often an unbiased representation of reality. A virtue of these investigations is the ability to rigidly control all known variables within an experiment. At the same time, this ability to exert control over an experiment can lead to bias. Also, the process of measurement itself is subject to observer bias or induced manipulation.

Definition of Nursing Practice by Operationalism

The need for nursing to provide the health care establishment and society with quantifiable measures and concrete definitions of nursing practice has led to the use of protocols and outcome criteria in the hope of demonstrating the value of nursing care. As previously discussed, use of the pragmatic method often leads to a tendency to attribute value to items by their function or outcome. This practice substitutes conceptually concrete measures for an individualized evaluation of each unique situation or occurrence. Although standardized protocols are advantageous as guidelines for care, the dogmatic application of them to all patient populations has serious implications for the health of the individual patient, as well as the health of the profession of nursing. Unfortunately, the type of measurable care defined in these protocols is often not representative of the complex array of behavioral, social, and biologic problem solving that was used prior to the laying on of hands.

As the ancient adage states, knowledge is power and is demonstrated by the synthesis of diverse pieces of data that leads to a rational conclusion. Representing a complex chain of knowledge solely by the use of protocols and outcome measures misrepresents the capacity of the individual nurse and the profession of nursing for intellectual achievement and complex problem solving. Although these methods provide a quantifiable measure of nursing care, they also may be perceived to represent an inability to be intellectually capable of using and applying complex knowledge. As social and scientific thought places a very high value on scientific process, the institution of these measures for conceptual thought results in a massive loss of power, prestige, and independent practice. As much of the current health care system operates on applied pragmatism, the profession of nursing is thereby relegated to a secondary status and is subject to a loss of power.

It is the very need of nurses to be valued by society as caregivers that has compelled the profession to use these narrow yet operationally clear measures to quantify the outcomes of nursing care. However, at this time not all of the facets of nursing care are measurable or quantifiable. Like the study of nonlinear dynamics and chaos, nursing practice deals not only with mechanistic physical systems but with as yet unquantifiable human behavior. Removing the variables of human behavior from these protocols has removed from societal consideration a major contribution of the nursing profession. Again, by ignoring phenomena solely due to our inability to quantify them reflects another way in which nursing is controlled by the prevailing societal value system. As we cannot quantify all the dimensions of nursing care, most care is invisible and does not exist to society.

Summary: Implications for Nursing

In nursing, as in common usage, the term pragmatic has become synonymous with "practical" rather than with the philosophical method of "pragmatism" or as a school of thought about knowledge. In the clinical setting, the term pragmatic is often used to praise those nurses who demonstrate an ability to be concerned with daily affairs unrestrained by theory or speculation. They are task oriented, efficient, and quickly complete the job at hand. Often, they are also described as practical and utilitarian (Guralnik, 1974). Operationally, the completion of the task at hand is the most important and only goal.

When such "practical" nurses are placed in the academic environment to pursue advanced education, they bring to the role of student the belief that only knowledge relating to the technical hands-on aspects of clinical practice is deemed worthy of attention and study. Unfortunately, this pattern of behavior is more closely allied to the functioning of the unionized assembly line worker than to that of an educated professional. Nursing practice based on such a model deprives the patient and family of the full range of nursing therapy and treatment by eliminating the psychosocial, cultural, and complex cognitive problem solving based in biobehavioral research that is the sine qua non of modern nursing. However, this narrow focus of intellectual functioning and role behavior may reflect the constraints of current institutional obsessions with financial status, cash flow, or the "bottom line." This practical approach looks toward a limited definition of the patient's future, focusing not on the very personal experience of illness surrounding the patient but on the outcome criteria of an efficient, task-oriented health care delivery system. Although efficiency of rote tasks within the constraints of a traditional 8-hour shift has always been promoted within the profession of nursing, it has never completely eclipsed the central tenet of nursing: alleviation of human misery due to illness and support of individuals to become autonomous.

References

Bender, A. D. (1990, October). Strategic plan needs focus, structure to aid vision. *Health Care Strategic Management*, pp. 12-15.

Buchler, J. (Ed.). (1955). *Philosophical writings of Peirce.* New York.

Dewey, J. (1931). *Philosophy and civilization.* New York: Peter Smith.

Gallie, W. B. (1952). *Peirce and pragmatism.* New York: Pelican Books.

Garfinkel, A., Spano, M. L., Ditto, W. L., & Weiss, J. N. (1992). Controlling cardiac chaos. *Science, 257*, 1230-1235.

Goetz, P. W. (Ed.). (1990). Philosophical schools and doctrines. In *Encyclopedia Britannica* (Vol. 25, pp. 645-649). Chicago: Encyclopedia Britannica.

Guralnik, D. B. (Ed.). (1974). *Webster's new world dictionary of the American language* (2nd college ed.). Cleveland, OH: Collins & World.

Hartshorne, C., Weiss, P., & Burks, A. W. (Ed.). (1931-1958). *The collected papers of Charles Sanders Peirce.* Cambridge, MA: Harvard University Press.

Hollander, S. F., Smith, M., & Barron, J. (1992). Cost reductions: Part 1. An operations improvement process. *Nursing Economics, 10*(5), 325-364.

James, W. (1975). *Pragmatism.* Cambridge, MA: Harvard University Press.

Kaplan, A. (1967). *The conduct of inquiry: Methodology for behavioral science.* Scranton, PA: Chandler.

Lewis, C. I. (1929). *Mind and the world order.* New York: Charles Scribner & Sons.

Omachonu, V. K., & Nanda, R. (1989). Measuring productivity: Outcome vs. output. *Nursing Management, 20*(4), 35-40.

Peirce, C. (1961). *The development of Peirce's philosophy.* Cambridge, MA: Harvard University Press.

Pool, R. (1989). Chaos theory: How big an advance. *Science, 245,* 26-29.

Prado, C. G. (1987). *The limits of pragmatism.* Atlantic Highlands, NJ: Humanities Press International.

Rorty, R. (1962). American pragmatism: Pierce, James, and Dewey. *International Journal of Ethics, 72,* 146-147.

Rorty, R. (1966). Charles Peirce and scholastic realism. *Philosophical Review, 75,* 116-119.

Rorty, R. (1971). Ayer's origins of pragmatism. *Philosophical Review, 80,* 96-100.

Wiener, P. (1973). Pragmatism. In *Dictionary of the history of ideas* (p. 433). New York: Scribner.

II

Revolutionary/Evolutionary Philosophy of Science

In the 1960s and 1970s, two significant challenges to the traditional empiricist philosophies of science appeared. These challenges have been referred to as historical critiques of empiricism, but will be referred to here as the revolutionary/evolutionary philosophies of science. The first of these revolutionary/evolutionary philosophies made its appearance with the work of Thomas Kuhn and his "paradigmatic" revolutionary text, *The Structure of Scientific Revolutions.* In her chapter, Jacquelyn Kegley explores the original text as well as Kuhn's more recent ideas. In her cogent review and critique of these ideas, Kegley explores how paradigmatic thought has influenced the discipline of philosophy, the scientific disciplines, and society in general. In the companion chapter, Barbara Riegel and coauthors use Kuhn's work as the basis for their own philosophy of nursing science. As such, this chapter provides an example of how one belief system can engender another. Larry Laudan, working in what could be called an evolutionary view of science, has also made a great contribution to the philosophy of science with his work, *Progress and Its Problems.* Sarah Fry examines and critiques Laudan's concept of science as a rational problem-solving activity. In her contribution, Cathy Ward explores how Laudan's philosophy, in conjunction with the work of Steven Toumlin, supports the understanding of the science and knowledge necessary in nursing administration. She describes how this philosophy gives direction to knowledge development within nursing administration, thus recognizing nursing administration as a valid area of scientific inquiry.

Science as Tradition and Tradition Shattering

Thomas Kuhn's Philosophy of Science

JACQUELYN ANN K. KEGLEY

Thomas Kuhn's (1962) *The Structure of Scientific Revolutions* (hereafter *SSR*), a book on the development of science via revolution, was itself a profoundly revolutionary document. It challenged many central elements of the prevailing philosophical view of "science," created a crisis within science's own self-understanding, provoked the redefinition of philosophy of science, history of science, and other related fields, and introduced a whole new vocabulary for those dealing with science and its alleged pursuit of knowledge. Anyone seriously concerned with analyzing the major characteristics of science, methods of scientific inquiry, and practice must come to grips with Kuhn's notion of "paradigm," "normal science," and "scientific revolutions." However, in understanding an analysis and description of Kuhn's thought one must acknowledge the tremendous body of critical literature stimulated by *SSR* that demonstrates a great deal of disagreement about Kuhn's central theses as well as alleged ambiguities in his statements and claims. A further complication in this regard is the fact that Kuhn, as analyst of science as an activity always in process, has himself continued to develop and explicate his views of the many issues raised by *SSR*. The most recent of these explications is his "Afterwords" (Kuhn, 1993) in *World Changes: Thomas Kuhn and the Nature of Science*, edited by Paul Horwich. The key publications in Kuhn's reflective process are indicated in the References section at the end of this chapter (Kuhn, 1962, 1963, 1970a, 1970b, 1970c, 1974, 1977, 1979, 1983a, 1983b, 1989, 1990).

What follows is my own "best" interpretation of Kuhn's central ideas, based on a review of his reflections and a fair amount of the critical literature. Fortunately, I also had the benefit of a new, definitive interpretation of Kuhn's work, namely, *Thomas Kuhn's Philosophy of Science* by Paul Hoyningen-Huene (1993).[1] In what follows, Kuhn's work is set first in the context of its challenge to the prevailing view of science and scientific development. Then the notion of "paradigm" and related concepts are discussed, followed by an explication of the distinctions between "normal" science and "prenormal" and "revolutionary" science. This leads to an analysis of "scientific revolution" with its issues of theory choice and incommensurability. A section on the question of "progress in science" and issues of rationality and relativism precedes a summary and criticisms.

The Context of Kuhn's Revolution

Kuhn's (1962) *SSR* caused such a stir in the intellectual world because it challenged a prevailing or "received view" about scientific development and the task of philosophy of science. This received view has been variously characterized and criticized,[2] but its main thrust was to carry out a logical analysis of science and to provide a rational reconstruction of scientific concepts and theories. It carried with it a foundationalist epistemology, arguing for scientific statements based on experience and confirmed by sensory data. Science's goal was *objective* knowledge intersubjectively verified and independent of individual opinion or preference. All scientific knowledge, on this view, consists of generalizations from experience that could ultimately be reduced to nonproblematic, directly observable phenomena or theoretical language assertions that were verifiable or at least testable.

Another important assumption of this prevailing view was that a sharp distinction could be made between the context of discovery (i.e., the processes leading up to the formulation of laws and theories, etc.) and the context of justification (e.g., the evidence and criteria used to warrant a theory). Further, it was claimed that universally valid methodological and epistemological standards existed by which science in general and the special sciences in particular could be evaluated.[3] In other words, there was only one method for science and following this method guaranteed science's objectivity. Science was *value free*. Further, from this viewpoint, philosophy of science was concerned only with the invariant characteristics of science. The history of science and its developmental features were unimportant. Only science's "finished products" were crucial, namely, "the end product of research, the careful statement in approved technical terms of something that had been empirically determined to be so" (McMullen, 1988, p. 15).

Another concern of this prevailing view in philosophy of science was intertheoretic reduction (i.e., the incorporation, as special cases, of earlier theories into later ones). The underlying assumption was that the history of science was a cumulative, rational process in which justified truth was built upon justified truth. Using the scientific (hypodeductive) method, science was amassing knowledge about the world. Science grows and progresses toward truth by a process of conjecture and refutation.

Kuhn's (1962) *SSR* represents a frontal attack on this view of science. In his book, science is seen in terms of periods of normal science dominated by a paradigm that dictates methodology and research projects, followed or interrupted by crises and scientific revolutions. Revolutions result in new theories or paradigms that are not cumulative additions to previous knowledge but, rather, replacements involving transformed concepts and ways of seeing the world. New theories are "incommensurably different" from the old theories they replace; there is no intertheoretic reduction. Kuhn also challenges the theoretical observation distinction of the received view. There are no "pure observables" to provide a foundation for scientific theory. Beliefs and theory play a fundamental role in perception; so-called facts are theory ladened. Further, given the fact that rival theories are incommensurable and that "meanings," "problems," and "questions" are dependent on theory, Kuhn believes that there is no unique way to evaluate theory, no one methodological rule to allow choice. Rather, theory choice involves a mixture of elements, including psychological and sociological facts; science does not proceed by conjecture and refutation. Kuhn's challenge, in fact, was to signal the end of the epoch of the "logical reconstruction of science."

Further, for Kuhn, the dynamic of scientific growth involves scientific communities, their beliefs, practices, and commitments, and not just individuals. Kuhn's emphasis on scientific knowledge as communal knowledge aligns him with contemporary feminist critiques. It also introduces sociological analysis and the question of "values." Kuhn (1970a) writes,

> It should be clear that the explanation must, in the final analysis, be psychological or sociological. It must, that is, be a description of a value system, an ideology, together with an analysis of the institutions through which that system is transmitted and enforced. Knowing what scientists value, we may hope to understand what problems they will undertake and what choices they will make in particular circumstances of conflict. (p. 21)

Finally, Kuhn does not see science as progressing toward some "truth" about the world as it really is. Rather, he has an instrumental view of the progress of science: namely, that science gains in precision and scope and in puzzle-solving ability (Kuhn, 1979). And, of course, for Kuhn the philosophy of science must be rooted in and responsible to its history. Because scientific progress is not cumulative, because there are "gains" and "losses" as science develops, one does not see "old science" as necessarily "bad science," or the past only as relevant to explaining the evolution of the presumed better contemporary scientific methods and concepts. Rather, one must display the historical integrity of past science in its own time. Indeed, something lost in the past may become a "gain" in the future. Kuhn (1979) writes, "The ontology of relativistic physics is, in significant respects, more like that of Aristotelian than of Newtonian physics" (p. 418).

The Paradigm Concept

At the heart of Kuhn's view of "science" is the notion of paradigm. There are undeniably some shifts in Kuhn's discussions of this notion, but the essential theses it embodies remain relatively stable. "Paradigm" places emphasis on professional consensus within a particular scientific community. It stands for the entire constellation of beliefs, values, and techniques shared by members of that community (*SSR*, p. 175). After 1969, Kuhn tended to use the term "disciplinary matrix" to encompass all aspects of the scientific consensus represented by the notion of paradigm. This term captures more clearly perhaps his conviction that analysis of scientific growth and revolution must be in terms of fundamental changes of point of view and practices of a concrete group of scientists in a given reality and at a given time (Kuhn, 1970a). It further is consonant with his belief that science progresses in terms of specialization and precision of problem solving (Kuhn, 1979, p. 418; 1993, p. 339).

"Paradigm" and "disciplinary matrix" embody the following elements. First, there are the symbolic generalizations, that is, the universal propositions regarded by the particular scientific community as the natural laws and/or fundamental equations of the operating theory(ies). These also contain the basic concepts of the paradigm (e.g., Newtonian "force" and "mass"). Models and/or metaphors are usually also an essential part of a paradigm. Examples are "Molecules of gas behave like tiny billiard balls in random motion," or "Atoms are like a miniature solar system." Models or metaphors have, says Kuhn, a property of open-endness, an inexplicitness. They play a crucial role in introducing new terms into the vocabulary of science as well as acquainting new generations of scientists with these concepts. They are guides to paradigm development as well as essential to stimulating the "similarity relations" essential to a paradigm's lexicon and to the way in which the paradigm's language "attaches to the world" (Kuhn, 1979, pp. 409, 414-415).

The lexicon of a paradigm is a notion that Kuhn developed after 1970. Kuhn (1993) defines a lexicon as "the module in which members of a speech community store the community's kind-terms" (p. 315). Kind-terms are essentially the categories by which a scientific community describes and generalizes about the world. They provide a set of learned expectations about the similarities and differences between objects and situations that populate the community's world. The lexicon is essentially the structuring of the "world" of a paradigm. It involves how things are "perceived," "categorized," and dealt with in terms of instrumentation and how they are related and how these relationships are formulized into laws. For example, the Aristotelian lexicon categorized free force (or motion) in terms of models of a "falling stone" or "spinning top" and forced motion in terms of a "hurled projectile." The Newtonian lexicon, on the other hand, saw free force as "movement in a straight line at constant speed," a categorization closely tied to Newton's first law of motion (Kuhn, 1990, p. 302).

The lexicon is the conceptual meaning of a paradigm, but it is closely tied both to ontolology and to scientific practice. The lexicon is learned in use, in scientific practice, in a community and is closely connected to another element of a paradigm, namely, the "exemplars," which are the shared examples that illustrate and direct the work of research, the practical solutions to problems, the fully specified instances of lab investigation that are described in textbooks on the specific achievements of the paradigms, such as Newton's deviation of the law of falling bodies, and the use of the spring balance to illustrate and embody Newton's third law as well as Hooke's law (Kuhn, 1990, p. 302f.).

The paradigm also involves value commitments to such criteria of theory evaluation as accuracy, scope, consistency, simplicity, and fruitfulness. Although "universal" in nature, these values, argues Kuhn, are articulated and prioritized in different ways by different scientific communities and even by the individuals within those communities. Their values are interrelated with and shaped by the other elements of the paradigm so that a community sees a particular situation, articulated in a particular way, as constituting a "scientific" problem and agrees that a particular way of dealing with the problem constitutes a "scientifically acceptable" solution to it. Thus what one paradigm sees as a scientific problem and/or solution worthy of pursuit will not be so judged by members of another paradigm community. In other words, different paradigms adopt different standards of excellence. Thus, for example, a value or criteria of excellence for a chemical theory before Lavoisier was to explain qualities such as color or texture as well as their changes. After Lavoisier, the ability to explain qualitative variation was no longer a criterion relevant to the evaluation of chemical theory (Kuhn, 1974, p. 364).

Incommensurability between paradigms has much to do with these various elements of a paradigm, but first we need to understand the role of paradigm in "normal" science.

Normal Science

Normal or "mature" science, is, for Kuhn, essentially paradigm-bound science (i.e., scientific practice is sustained by a broad-based community consensus of foundational issues). In other words, there are accepted symbolic generalizations, models, values, and exemplars and an implict lexicon and ontology. Normal science is predicated on "the assumption that the scientific community knows what the world is like" (*SSR,* p. 149). The practitioners of a mature, scientific specialty are committed to a paradigm-based way of regarding and investigating nature. The main task of normal science is puzzle solving undertaken with a deep commitment to the paradigm and aimed at bringing that paradigm "into closer and closer agreement with nature" (Kuhn, 1963, p. 360). The effort is directed, first of all, to articulating the paradigm, rendering it more precise, applying it to areas where it is assumed to work but to which it has not yet been applied. Some have described the activities of normal science as "mopping up details."

Normal science has a certain "dogmatic tenor" because calling the paradigm into question is not appropriate. If failure in experimentation occurs, it usually reflects back on the scientist's inability to provide a solution. Normal science is made possible, in fact, says Kuhn, by a form of training and education that promotes highly convergent modes of thought. Textbooks highlight the agreed-on exemplars and teach the implicit lexicon and model. Students receive, says Kuhn (1963), a "relatively dogmatic initiation into a previously established problem-solving tradition" (p. 351). Through such an education, students gain access to the implicit and explicit knowledge of the field and to the "world of the paradigm." They also gain an extraordinarily efficient mastery of the techniques employed in finding and solving the problems of normal science.

Indeed, contrary to Popper and others, Kuhn does not see normal science as "bad" science but believes it to be essential to the advance of science. Nature, says Kuhn, cannot be explored at random. There is great heuristic value to scientific belief and conviction. Indeed, there is scientific progress within the paradigm as it is perfected and expanded. The value of normal science is also seen in terms of "prenormal" science, a stage of science in which there is competition between various schools of thought. As a result, argues Kuhn, research problems are not unequivocally identified because there is no guide, no examplars. In prenormal science, there is little if any progress and much repetition and reiteration of efforts.

The valuable aspects of normal science and its contrast to prenormal science have led a number of theorists to argue that paradigm achievement is necessary in science to make scientific achievement possible. It is claimed, for example, that the social sciences are not yet "genuine" sciences because paradigm consensus has not yet been achieved. Others have found such arguments fallacious or misinterpretations of Kuhn's work (Roth, 1984). Some believe that appeal to "paradigm bound" as the key to science and its advancement is dangerous (e.g., that it encourages totalitarianism and intolerance).

Kuhn also recognizes a paradox in the dogmatic tenor of normal science, namely, that although fundamental to productive research it suggests that preconception and resistance to innovation rather than exploration and discovery is the rule rather than the exception in scientific development. Scientific orthodoxy seems to be an important part of science. Dolby (1980) extensively researched the evidence for such orthodoxy and argues that it emerged not only to promote the generation of new knowledge but also to allow the assimilation of science into the rest of society (p. 202). Dolby argues that orthodoxy has provided quality control (i.e., it prevents fraud and quacks claiming scientific validity) but also has constituted "restricted practice, namely, it has prevented the circulation of work later recognized as important" (p. 214).

Scientific Revolutions

Whatever our judgment on the function of dogma in scientific development, Kuhn is clear that the paradigm-binding nature of normal science is an essential part of the advancement of science through revolutions. The very strength and unanimity of the paradigm provides

the individual scientist with an immensely sensitive detector of the trouble spots from which significant innovations of fact and theory are almost inevitably induced. Therefore, although a quasi-dogmatic commitment is, on the one hand, a source of resistance and controversy, it is also instrumental in making the sciences the most consistently revolutionary of all human activities. (Kuhn, 1963, p. 349)

Revolutions begin with a "crisis" within a paradigm. Recognizing that something is fundamentally wrong with the paradigm upon which they work, scientists will seek new articulations not considered permissible earlier. Out of the ferment of this revolutionary period, a new paradigm will emerge. It is truly "revolutionary" because a new paradigm is a conceptual transformation, a modification of lexical structure, a change in worldview. What is involved is a fundamental shift in scientific practice; new value configurations occur; and the meaning of "scientific activity" itself changes.

To describe the profound change in a scientific revolution, Kuhn speaks of the incommensurability of paradigms. This incommensurability has several aspects. First, the set of scientific problems and solutions changes. Answers or questions once considered central may now be considered trivial or irrelevant, and questions and solutions that did not exist appear. Second, there is a fundamental change in lexicon; there is transformation of both concepts and procedures, or expectations of behavior and relationships. Symbolic generalizations undergo changes that new models or metaphors develop. As for meaning change, it can be both extensional and intentional—for example, in the transition from the Ptolemaic to the Copernican view, "earth" changed both its class and its attributes—and because the lexicon mediates the relation of the conceptual structure to the world, the change in the structure of the lexicon brings about a "change in the world."

Further, because observation and perception are theory or paradigm dependent (i.e., the terms that occur in both paradigms are a function of the paradigm in which they appear), there is incommensurability between paradigms in that there is untranslatability. There is no neutral observation language into which each paradigm may be translated; there is "no language into which at least the empirical consequences of both can be translated without loss or change" (Kuhn, 1970b, p. 266).

However, Kuhn did not intend for incommensurability to signal, as many critics imply, "incomparability." Paradigms do deal with the same "object domain," and some empirical predictions can be compared. Further, although it is very difficult, scientists can become bilingual;

that is, they can learn the "language" of the new paradigm. Whatever one finally decides on the issues of incommensurability and comparability, however, it should be clear, for Kuhn, that revolutions imply discontinuity and losses within the development of science. Science is not epistemically cumulative. The new paradigm is not compatible with previous existing knowledge; rather than envelopment of the old in the new, there is replacement.

Theory choice, for Kuhn, then is not merely a mode of methodological assessment or "falsification by direct comparison with nature" (*SSR*, p. 77) but, rather, a combination of elements (e.g., faith, value considerations, argument, and comparison) as well as dependent on individual differences. The first adherents of the new theory must have "faith" that the new theory will succeed with problems where the old theory failed; yet there is also argument and debate. In fleshing out the new paradigm, these first adherents must eventually convince the scientific community of the promise of this new view. "Persuasion," in the sense of argument and counterargument, is involved, and to use this word, says Kuhn, is *not* to suggest that there are not many good reasons for choice. Scientific values, especially those related to the task of solving as many research problems as possible, are also involved. Thus it must be apparent to the scientific community that the new theory is able to solve the problems brought on by the crisis with greater accuracy than the old. "Fruitfulness" is another value that might be evoked, that is, the ability of the new theory to predict phenomena that from the perspective of the older theory are unexpected. The "value" or "aesthetic" judgments involved should not, as critics argue, suggest that the decision at issue is *necessarily* irrational or arational (Kuhn, 1970b, p. 262; Machan, 1977, p. 362). Above all, for Kuhn, there are no universal, mechanical rules of choice (Kuhn, 1977, p. 331; *SSR*, p. 200). Criteria for choosing vary with field of application and with epoch (Kuhn, 1977, p. 335), and the criteria for choosing are always imprecise (Kuhn, 1977, pp. 321-322; *SSR*, pp. 199, 205).

Is There Progress in Science?

As indicated above, Kuhn denies progress in science if it means drawing closer to the truth about the world as it really is. He believes the history of science speaks against ontological convergence (e.g.,

Aristotle's ontology is closer to Einstein's than is Newton's). Further, Kuhn believes it is meaningless to talk about what is really there beyond all theory. Language, or lexicon, for Kuhn, structures the world. There is a "phenomenal world" specific to a given community; that community is the constituting agent for this world. Kuhn speaks of a "reluctant pluralism of phenomenal or professional worlds." However, he does also acknowledge a resistance of the inaccessible "environment" or "thing in itself" world, which provides limits to our conceptual structures and explains anomalies and crises. This spatiotemporal purely object-sided environment is somehow "causally efficacious," so that the "phenomenal world" of a paradigm is, so to speak, determined jointly by nature and the paradigm. However, although "we face the effects of these (concrete properties of the world-in-itself) in the resistance the world offers to our epistemic efforts, we are not in a position to grasp this resistance as it is in itself" (Hoyningen-Huene, 1993, p. 270).

Progress in science, then, is instrumental for Kuhn, involving an increased ability and precision in problem solving. Doppelt (1978) has characterized Kuhn's view as a "gradualist view of scientific development," namely, one that denies that progress necessarily occurs in major stages or parts of science, but that scientific development "as a whole may ultimately satisfy a criterion of progress" (p. 721). This interpretation may or may not faithfully reflect Kuhn's own view. It depends on the exact meaning of the word "progress."

This issue will continue to be debated. However, I believe Kuhn's resistance to the notion of "progress" could be developed in context of the many discussions of whether there is technological progress. The answer may depend on the goals and values one believes relevant to judging the issue (e.g., expediency and efficiency or human development and good). It just may not be the case that knowledge and truth will always receive the highest priority.

Work Yet to Be Done

Kuhn's work is seminal and cannot be ignored by those who wish to analyze science or to do science. Clearly, the notions of paradigm, lexicon, revolution, and incommensurability contain much truth and provide guidance to our understanding of science and of scientific development. Kuhn has disturbed our complacency about science as an autonomous, preeminent objective, value-free, ultimately rational enterprise. Rather, we can now see science as a fundamentally human creative enterprise, an essentially human form of *praxis*, a way of perceiving, understanding, and acting upon the world. Kuhn makes clear also the essentially communal nature of science by focusing on the practice of specific scientific communities. His work opens the door to a recognition that knowledge seeking, although done by individual scientists, is always a communal enterprise, socially informed, pragmatically oriented, and partially conditioned by its historical and communal context. Those interested in scientific knowledge seeking need to be necessarily involved with history, sociology, and social psychology.

Indeed, Kuhn's emphasis on science as a "communal activity," moves us, as the feminists and others have recognized (Nelson, 1990), in the direction of undermining the essentially individualist, rationalistic bias of traditional epistemology as well as social, political, and moral philosophy. It allows us to explore the role that "values," including those related to social/political views of "cognitive authority," play in what was regarded as a completely "value free" activity. It allows us to explore naturalistic epistemology (i.e., the attempt to discover how the beliefs we have are acquired) as well as to examine ways that scientific language, including models, reflect social and cultural contexts, such as the use of linear, hierarchical causal models in biology (Bleier, 1984). If science is a form of human praxis, among others, it allows further exploration of science and practice disciplines, such as nursing and medicine.[4]

However, although seeing science in its human social and historical context is important, a perusal of the critical literature on Kuhn tells us that we need to also be concerned about strongly relativistic overtones of his work as well as sensitive to the profound threats to notions of rationality his theses seem to pose. I do not believe Kuhn's intent is to embrace the anarchistic proliferation of theories view of Feyerabend. He clearly believes the dogmatic overtones of normal science, the "voicing consensus," to be essential to scientific progress while recognizing the possible and actual inhibiting force this can be. Kuhn's views require us to struggle with carefully balancing necessary constraints to the scientific enterprise along with empowering creativity and innovation. Kuhn believes in constraints provided both by nature and by values essential to the enterprise of science, namely, accuracy, fruitfulness, and simplicity. If these values fail or are not operative, argues Kuhn, then the form of human life in Western culture known as "science" also fails. These value constraints, however, allow for individual variability; each member applies values of the shared paradigm differently, and thus creativity and dissent are also part of normal science as well as of revolutionary science. Again, Kuhn challenges prevailing notions of a radical fact/value distinction and of values as necessarily irrational and subjective. As Holcomb (1989) has suggested, Kuhn's work on "value judgments" in science stimulates and requires work on the interrelationship of philosophy of science and moral philosophy.

As for the constraints of nature, we find Kuhn's (1979) Kantianism "without things-in-themselves" and "with changing categories of mind" (p. 419) less than satisfactory. I would prefer clearer emphasis on the pressures and contraints of "reality." To my mind, a good alternative is a Peircean-type realism that stresses (a) fallibility, uncertainty, losses, and gains in seeking knowledge and (b) the crucial role of community but that holds science to be moving toward truth and a picture of reality. With Peirce, I believe science, in its puzzle-solving and revolutionary activity, somehow works; a fit, perhaps not perfect, with reality occurs. In his most recent reflection, Kuhn (1993) suggests this when he writes,

> Puzzle-solving is one of the families of practices that has arisen during that (human) evolution, and what it produces is knowledge of nature. Those who proclaim that no interest-driven practice can properly be identified as the rational pursuit of knowledge make a profound and consequential mistake. (p. 339).

Notes

1. In Hoyningen-Huene's (1993) book, Kuhn writes in the Preface, "I could not have asked for an interlocutor more patient, more independent, or more concerned to get both detail and overall direction right. Readers who care about resolving the puzzles to be found in my writings will be in his debt for a long time to come. No one, myself included, speaks with as much authority about the nature and developments of my ideas" (p. xi).

2. For an excellent overview of the "received view" and the developments leading to its demise, see Suppe's (1977) "Afterword."

3. Burian (1977) thus aptly characterizes this received view of philosophy of science as "logicism."

4. See Zheng (1988) for an interesting illustration of Kuhnian incommensurability using Western and Chinese medicine as the two paradigms.

References

Bleier, R. (1984). Science and gender: A critique of biology and its theories on women. New York: Pergamon Press.

Burian, R. D. (1977). More than a marriage of convenience: On the history and philosophy of science. *Philosophy of Science, 44,* 1-42.

Dolby, R. G. A. (1980). Controversy and consensus in the growth of scientific knowledge. *Nature and System, 2,* 199-218.

Doppelt, G. (1978). Kuhn's epistemological relativism: An interpretation and defense. *Inquiry, 21,* 33-86.

Holcomb, H. R., III. (1989). Interpreting Kuhn's paradigm—Choice as objective value judgment. *Metaphilosophy, 20*(1), 51-67.

Hoyningen-Huene, P. (1993). *Thomas Kuhn's philosophy of science* (A. T. Levine, Trans.). Chicago: University of Chicago Press.

Kuhn, T. (1962). *The structure of scientific revolutions.* Chicago: University of Chicago Press.

Kuhn, T. (1963). The function of dogma in scientific research. In A. C. Crombie (Ed.), *Scientific change, historical studies in the intellectual, social and technical conditions for scientific discovery and technical invention, from antiquity to the present* (pp. 347-369). London: Heinemann.

Kuhn, T. (1970a). Logic of discovery or psychology of research? In I. Lakatos & A. Musgrave (Eds.), *Criticism and the growth of knowledge* (pp. 231-278). Cambridge: Cambridge University Press.

Kuhn, T. (1970b). Reflections on my critics. In I. Lakatos & A. Musgrave (Eds.), *Criticism and the growth of knowledge* (pp. 1-23). Cambridge: Cambridge University Press.

Kuhn, T. (1970c). Postscript—1969. In T. Kuhn, *The structure of scientific revolutions* (2nd ed.). Chicago: University of Chicago Press.

Kuhn, T. (1974). Second thoughts on paradigms. In F. Suppe (Ed.), *The structure of scientific theories* (pp. 459-482). Urbana: University of Illinois Press. (Also appears in Kuhn's *Essential tension,* 1977, pp. 293-319)

Kuhn, T. (1977). Objectivity, value judgment and theory choice. In T. Kuhn, *Essential tension* (pp. 320-339). Chicago: University of Chicago Press.

Kuhn, T. (1979). Metaphor in science. In A. Ortony (Ed.), *Metaphor and thought* (pp. 409-419). Cambridge: Cambridge University Press.

Kuhn, T. (1983a). Commensurability, comparability, communicability. In P. D. Asquith & T. Nickles (Eds.), *Proceedings of the 1982 Biennial Meeting of the Philosophy of Science Association* (pp. 669-688). East Lansing, MI: Philosophy of Science Association.

Kuhn, T. (1983b). Rationality and theory choice. *Journal of Philosophy, 80,* 563-570.

Kuhn, T. (1989). Possible worlds in history of science. In S. Allen (Ed.), *Possible worlds in humanities, arts, and sciences* (pp. 49-51). Berlin: de Gruyter.

Kuhn, T. (1990). Dubbing and redubbing: The vulnerability of rigid designation. In C. W. Savage (Ed.), *Scientific theories* (Minnesota Studies in Philosophy of Science, vol. 14, pp. 298-318). Minneapolis: University of Minnesota Press.

Kuhn, T. (1993). Afterwords. In P. Horwich (Ed.), *World changes: Thomas Kuhn and the nature of science* (pp. 311-341). Cambridge: MIT Press.

Machan, T. R. (1977). Kuhn, paradigm choice and the arbitrariness of aesthetic criteria in science. *Theory and Decision, 8,* 361-362.

McMullen, E. (1988). *Construction and constraint.* Notre Dame, IN: Notre Dame University Press.

Nelson, L. H. (1990). *Who knows? From Quine to feminist epistemology.* Philadelphia: Temple University Press.

Roth, P. A. (1984). Who needs paradigms? *Metaphilosophy, 15*(3-4), 225-238.

Suppe, F. (Ed.). (1977). *The structure of scientific theories* (2nd ed.). Urbana: University of Illinois Press.

Zheng, L. (1988). Incommensurability and scientific rationality. *International Studies in Philosophy of Science, 2,* 227-236.

Suggested Readings

Calapietro, V. M. (1987). Toward a more comprehensive conception of human reason. *International Philosophical Quarterly, 28,* 282-298.

Grandy, R. E. (1983). Incommensurability: Kinds and causes. *Philosophica, 32,* 7-24.

Kegley, J. A. K. (1989). History and philosophy of science: Necessary partners or merely roommates? In T. Z. Lavine & V. Tejera (Eds.), *History and anti-history in philosophy* (pp. 237-255). New York: Kluwer Academic.

Kegley, J. A. K. (1992). Technology as creativity and embodiment: A new critical view. In *Proceedings of the Institute of Liberal Studies: Science Technology and Religious Ideas III* (pp. 11-19). Latham, MD: University Press of America.

Moving Beyond

A Generative Philosophy of Science

BARBARA RIEGEL, ANNA OMERY,

EVELYN CALVILLO, NAIEMA GABER ELSAYED,

PATRICIA LEE, PAMELA SHULER, AND

BONNIE ELLEN SIEGEL

Nursing science is a science in search of its philosophical foundation. Evidence of the intensity of this search is apparent in nursing's journals. Articles that propose various philosophies of science for nursing from empiricism to critical theory abound (Allen, 1985; Norbeck, 1987). Nursing seems intent on finding an existing philosophy of science and adopting it as it stands as the philosophical foundation for the discipline.

AUTHORS' NOTE: The contents of this chapter were previously published in *Image* and are adapted here with permission.

The fact that no single, dominant philosophy of science has yet prevailed gives evidence that an appropriate philosophical foundation for nursing science has not been found. If nursing continues to search for a philosophy to adopt, we will always be following and falling somewhere behind the philosophical development occurring in other disciplines. It is our opinion that a philosophy of science for nursing must come from nurses. Any philosophy adopted must be consistent with nursing's philosophy of practice, as the aim of nursing science is not the development of knowledge for knowledge's sake; nursing science is symbiotic with nursing practice.

Nurses must begin to critically examine, articulate, and share their current beliefs about practice and science. This examination may result in a new vision of science, one that relates to practice. Such a vision will be a proactive rather than a reactive one.

This chapter describes a philosophy of science, the generative philosophy of science, and its relationship to nursing practice. The generative philosophy of science was so named because to generate means to bring into being, to form, to develop. This meaning is consistent with the goal of this philosophy as facilitating growth among practice disciplines for which previously articulated philosophies of science may not be adequate.

From Whence We Came

At least four major schools of thought have influenced (covertly or overtly) nursing's philosophy of science: logical positivism and the paradigmatic, evolutionary, and feminist schools.

Proponents of logical positivism view science as a body of knowledge that is value free, independent of the scientist, and obtained using an objective method (Kemeny, 1959; Silva & Rothbart, 1984). The goal of logical positivism is to explain, to predict, and, according to recent feminist theory (Keller, 1985), to control or dominate nature. Formalized theory that is either true or false, subject to empirical observation, and capable of being reduced into existing scientific theories achieves the goals of science most ably.

As a young science, nursing emulated the more established disciplines, such as physiology, that ascribed to the logical positivistic model. As Gortner (1983) pointed out, "What had worked for one science was expected to work for another" (p. 3). Although early advocates of logical positivism now acknowledge that it is inappropriate in isolation (Jacox & Webster, 1986), logical positivism continues to influence what is condoned in nursing as "scientific" knowledge. For instance, the subject matter deemed appropriate for examination by scientists is that which is objective and empirical. Acceptable methods for knowledge generation are those that are traditional, orthodox, and preferably experimental (Jacox & Webster, 1986). The influence of subjectivity on the choice of researchable questions and the interpretation of results must be denied. However, acceptance of purely quantitative, experimental research methods to the exclusion of qualitative and descriptive methods excludes knowledge important for the profession (Munhall, 1982).

In the United States, logical positivism predominated until the 1960s when Thomas Kuhn (1970) introduced the paradigmatic conception of science. Kuhn's philosophical view of science was the result of the failure of deductive methodology to achieve the goals of prediction and control in the human sciences. The deductive method limited researchable phenomena and disregarded the influence of values on science.

According to the paradigmatic view, normal science is an orderly, functional process firmly based on one or more past scientific achievements that a particular scientific community acknowledges. Normal science is a dynamic process interrupted by explosive, intermittent crises that revolutionize science and change the direction of growth within and across disciplinary paradigms (Kuhn, 1970). Values and beliefs are acknowledged as integral to the aim of discovering, understanding, and explaining phenomena.

Although Kuhn introduced significant ideas and important contributions to the conception of science, problems with the paradigmatic view existed. Science and other major concepts such as paradigm, crisis, and revolution were never fully defined. For example, Masterman (1970) noted that paradigm is used by Kuhn (1970) in 22 different ways. Although Kuhn's view should be valued for acknowledging dynamism in science and allowing for values and beliefs in the process, his vagueness and vacillating, contradictory stance published 7 years later (Kuhn, 1977) limits usefulness of his philosophy.

Evolutionary philosophers, such as Laudan (1977), fathered some of the most recent philosophies of science advocated by nurses (Gorenberg, 1983; Ramos, 1987). The evolutionary philosophy views science as an economical, problem-solving process that advances in an orderly, progressive fashion. The impetus for this evolutionary process is based soundly in societal need; rational knowledge gained through problem solving is used to help humankind. The evolutionary philosophy of science is appealing, but Laudan's (1977) focus on problem solving seemed inconsistent with nursing's practice perspective on health maintenance and problem prevention.

The impact of society and history on conceptions of science is also evident in articles supporting feminism (Bunting & Campbell, 1990; Hagell, 1989) and critical theory perspectives (Allen, 1985; Thompson, 1985) that now appear in the nursing literature. The influences of gender, culture, society, and shared history are essential integral components of science in these philosophies, making them appealing because many of these concepts are consistent with nursing's worldview. However, these philosophies still are borrowed, a process that inhibits nursing's efforts to describe its own unique beliefs regarding science.

It is evident that no one philosophy represents nursing in its complexity and richness. The poor fit between existing philosophies of science and practice disciplines, such as nursing, has caused the values of these young sciences to be questioned (Benner & Wrubel, 1989). Nursing is presently generating knowledge at a pace unequaled in its history. However, nurses continue to question the relevancy and appropriateness of that knowledge and the methods used to generate it (Clarke & Yaros, 1988; Phillips, 1988). It is time for nursing to examine its science with the goal of articulating a philosophical position consistent with the beliefs and values of this practice discipline.

The generative philosophy of science was developed as a first step toward meeting such a goal. The philosophy presented here is the result of two different yet complementary processes that took place over two years. The first process included review of current nursing theories and competing philosophies of science. Nursing practice was critically examined against that review as a framework for our beliefs about a philosophy of science. The resulting generative philosophy of science was influenced by all the philosophies previously described but predominately that of Kuhn (1970). Using the paradigmatic philosophy as a base, we clarified obscurities, expanded concepts, added original ideas, and borrowed some found in other philosophies of science and theoretical papers. For instance, the importance of linking research methods with disciplinary values was borrowed from Laudan

(1977). Silva and Rothbart (1984) note that the case study rather than an experimental design with "built-in reductionism" (p. 4) should be used to research holism. Issues of gender, culture, history, and societal influence were taken from the feminist view.

The second process was a critical examination of our beliefs regarding major concepts such as science, discipline, matrix, nursing, and nursing practice. External review of earlier drafts of this chapter also assisted in clarifying inconsistencies and ambiguity. The product presented here is the result of these processes.

A Generative Philosophy of Nursing Science

The constituents of the generative philosophy of science are society, disciplines, and science, all of which exist as open interdependent systems. Science is unique knowledge that results from a distinct procedure. The aim of science is the discovery, description, understanding, explanation, prediction, and verification of empirical knowledge. Science exists within disciplines that are organized and structured by matrices. Disciplines are found within societies. The concepts of society, disciplines, and science are not unique to this philosophy. However, the definitions and interrelationships are developed in a manner consistent with contemporary values and beliefs of nursing.

Definitions

Society is a term meant to refer to all people and all cultures. Within societies are groups of individuals who share common traditions, institutions, and interests. Societies are characterized by the beliefs and the values of the members of those groups. All philosophies of science address society as the backdrop against which science occurs. In the generative philosophy of science, however, society has a major role: to reflect the important influence of values and beliefs on science.

Society maintains a reciprocal relationship with science and disciplines. Society advances science through the respect and attention accorded disciplinary scientists based on perceived social need and relevance; science influences society through education and the scientific products generated. Disciplines are influenced by the social relevance and values of society (Donaldson & Crowley, 1978); society provides respect and monetary reward to disciplinary members based on the degree of value accorded their contribution to society. A society sustains disciplines and sciences that follow the mandate of that society's beliefs and values. For instance, whereas those who practice palmistry espouse it as a science, mainstream society does not support it as such.

A case could be made that the science of nursing has had trouble developing because of its relationship with society's beliefs and values. Reverby (1984) noted in her historical review of American nursing that nurses have been "ordered to care" in a society that does not value caring.

Disciplines are branches of knowledge organized by matrices. The uniqueness of a discipline stems from the matrix, which is a combination of structure and tradition. Individuals who practice from a discipline hold a similar world view of perspective that is the result of the matrix. The uniqueness of a discipline stems from its perspective, not empirical findings (Donaldson & Crowley, 1978). The term matrix is used rather than paradigm (Kuhn, 1970) or research tradition (Laudan, 1977) to communicate that what binds a group together is its unique perspective.

A matrix is a combination of structure and tradition that lends a unique identity to the discipline. The structure gives organization to the matrix; tradition provides the content. The structure or organization of the disciplinary matrix determines the amount, relationship, and specific ratio of each type of knowledge allowed to constitute the discipline. Traditions include ethical, personal, aesthetic (or artful nursing practice), and scientific knowledge.

The disciplinary matrix, with its unique structure and tradition, both differentiates nursing from other disciplines and determines which phenomena will be recognized as legitimate areas of concern. Use of the disciplinary matrix in practice is influenced by the cultural beliefs and values of society. Although nurses worldwide would probably identify person, health, environment, and nursing as key constructs (Flaskerud & Halloran, 1980), research and practice differ, based on values (Gortner, 1983), health care needs of the society, population characteristics, access to alternate providers, and education, to name a few. The strong influence of societal traditions may cause the empirical knowledge of the discipline to be viewed differently, resulting in varying interpretations of the matrix.

Disciplines develop as the result of creative thinking by a group of individuals. The result of this creative thinking is the matrix that cements together disciplinary and practice members of the group. Individuals promote activity within a discipline through the use of creative and scientific methods designed to address phenomena of concern drawn from the matrix. Nursing has begun to identify phenomena of concern including wellness, quality of life, and adherence, to name a few.

Science is a unique kind of knowledge. Science is generated by the human application of a rigorous, distinct procedure or method; that method is, in itself, a specific type of scientific knowledge. Disciplinary members interpret the knowledge generated by scientific procedures through their specific matrix.

The knowledge that is science is empirical knowledge. Empirical knowledge is those data available to the individual through the senses. This knowledge is intersubjective in nature in that it is capable of being agreed on by rational human beings. This definition differs from that of logical positivism with its emphasis on objective knowledge that exists independent of the knower (Kemeny, 1959).

Empirical knowledge is composed of individual, specific data that are organized into concepts and theories. Concepts are abstractions describing specific data or phenomena; theories describe the organization or processes by which concepts relate. Knowledge is dynamic but not linear, evolutionary, cumulative, or necessarily progressive as mandated by logical positivism (Popper, 1979).

The scientific procedure, which is itself knowable, is a rational, purposeful, complex human activity requiring forethought, planning, and intent to generate new knowledge. This procedure uses a variety of systematic, rigorous methods with the aim of discovery, description, understanding, explanation, prediction, and verification of knowledge. Science generates, integrates, and reflects values derived from history, tradition, culture, and society (Keller, 1985). A dynamic science incorporates the influence of, and causes an influence on, individual and societal beliefs and values. This assumption is consistent with Kuhn (1970) and Laudan (1977) but in direct opposition to logical positivists such as Popper (1979), who states that science is a product that is independent of the scientist and of societal value.

Defining the scientific procedure as rational and purposeful is consistent with logical positivism, a stance opposed by some (Benner & Wrubel, 1979) as denying the subject's connection to his or her situation. However, it is asserted that the scientific process must be reasonable and logical (i.e., rational) if understanding is to progress. Further, acknowledging the aims of discovery and description allows for a far wider variety of research methods than allowed by logical positivism. Nurses concerned with the biological, psychological, and social components of patients must have the flexibility to choose a research method consistent with the question asked. Experimental methods may be ideal for biological questions (e.g., what is the effect of toileting on myocardial oxygen consumption?); however, ethnography may be preferred for describing a Hispanic woman's response to labor and delivery. Control is not incorporated as an aim of science, although it is acknowledged as an essential component of experimental research methods.

Relationships Among Society, Disciplines, and Science

A reciprocal relationship exists among society, science, and disciplines. Science exists within disciplines, and disciplines exist within society. A discipline is larger than the science that it structures. Disciplines differ in the proportion of the various types of knowledge. Mature disciplines that hold predominately scientific knowledge are known as scientific entities. Disciplines that have little formal scientific knowledge may exist as arts with the potential for becoming sciences. For instance, chiropractic practice consists primarily of personal and artful practice knowledge, as little formal chiropractic science has been developed. The nursing discipline remains predominately artful practice knowledge, but the proportion of the discipline that is scientific knowledge is steadily increasing.

The empirical questions suitable for investigation by disciplinary scientists are constantly negotiated based on societal and matrix beliefs and values. In this process, other types of knowledge are determined either to be or not to be suitable for scientific investigation within a particular disciplinary matrix.

Science: A Human Activity

DISCIPLINARY MEMBERS

All disciplines are composed of varying and unique proportions of practitioners and scientists. Practitioners in disciplines such as nursing include both technicians and professionals. We believe that each role (technician, professional, scientist) contributes an essential component to a discipline as complex as nursing.

Technicians in nursing necessarily become experts in practice knowledge. As practice experts, they bring unrecognized data to the attention of other disciplinary members so that new information can be used for the good of society. The professional acts as a link between the technician and the scientist by identifying areas of research for the scientist and by sharing and interpreting research results with the technician. Scientists are prepared to use rigorous systematic research processes to achieve the goal of contributing scientific knowledge to the discipline. The scientist uses the scientific procedure to generate, examine, and interpret data entering the discipline through practitioners, with the aim being to discover, describe, understand, explain, predict, and verify knowledge within the discipline and thereby contributing to society.

Nurse scientists educated at the doctoral level are responsible for knowledge development in a science barely out of the embryonic stage (Carper, 1978). This knowledge must have clinical relevance to be useful to the technicians and professionals in clinical practice and to society in general. Most nurse scientists have a history of practice experience that provides a sound grasp of the types of knowledge found within the discipline. A history of nursing practice facilitates the exploration of useful questions. Nurses often practice at more than one level; a scientist may discover knowledge and also be a professional who applies it. Use of this unique dual perspective helps ensure that knowledge is generated that is useful to disciplinary members and society.

One question generated by this model is what qualifies a particular investigation as fitting into the discipline of nursing? A scientist educated within one discipline is not necessarily conducting research in that discipline unless she or he is studying phenomena pertinent to the disciplinary members, that is, as viewed through the matrix of the discipline. Conversely, a scientist educated in one discipline can conduct research within another. However, education in one discipline and the conduct of science within another can result in disruptive or irrelevant scientific products. For example, a few nurses educated in related disciplines such as psychology or physiology who return to nursing can offer new theories and research methods that may enhance nursing. However, a large number of nurses socialized into a different discipline during intensive years of education may no longer value or even recognize nursing's disciplinary matrix or may not be interested in studying the phenomena with which nurses are concerned.

ACTIVITIES OF SCIENTISTS

The scientific members of a discipline must participate in two types of activities: concrete and conceptual. *Concrete activities* consist of actual human actions, which may range from qualitative inquiry to laboratory research conducted using traditional experimental methods. Concrete activity is a necessary but insufficient condition for science. That is, concrete activity is necessary to verify conceptual activity, and indeed, cannot exist without conceptual activity.

Conceptual activity is the essential activity of scientists and acts as the gate that allows specific information or data to enter the science. Conceptual activity performs as a discriminator. Information that enters the discipline has little to great potential for being scientific knowledge. The scientist decides which of the empirical data will enter the discipline by using conceptual activity.

Once data enter a discipline through its members they are investigated by scientists in an attempt to identify concepts. Knowledge generated within a discipline is organized through conceptual activity as theories that account for or characterize some phenomena (Andreoli & Thompson, 1977). These theories ultimately may result in law, or accepted reality, that are used by society.

Data determined by conceptual activity of the scientist to be anomalous for one discipline may feed another discipline or result in new or differently focused disciplines. Data originally entering one discipline may be discarded only to be assimilated by another discipline. For example, data from nonadherent patients have traditionally been judged as merely irritating to medical scientists, whereas nurses and psychologists have assimilated those data as important to their disciplines.

New or differently focused disciplines result from an accumulation of anomalies that subsequently are addressed by a group of individuals from within or from without the discipline (Kuhn, 1970). Data judged by most members as anomalous may be seen as innovative and provocative by a subgroup that moves the discipline in a new direction. For instance, when Rogers (1980) incorporated the concept of energy fields into the theory of unitary man, this was a new and controversial perspective for nurses. Disciplinary members may differ in opinions regarding what data should be considered anomalous and what should not. Acceptance of diverse data within a single disciplinary matrix is understandable because perceptions of data are influenced by individual, disciplinary, and societal values and beliefs.

Challenges for the Future

The generative philosophy of science is not presented as a finished product. Certain areas still require clarification or possibly even reconceptualization. The hope is that consumers of the model will not use those areas of concern as an excuse to prematurely abandon the philosophy. Rather, the desire is that the philosophy be used as a starting point for discussions about what belief system constitutes an appropriate foundation for science in disciplines such as nursing.

For this model to function as a necessary and sufficient philosophical foundation for the science of nursing, discussions will have to focus on answering questions in at least two broad areas: the relationship of disciplines to one another and clarification of concepts within disciplines.

Although the preceding discussion attempted to address the relationship of the disciplines to society, little of it focused on the relationships among disciplines. Questions raised in our discussion but left unresolved are the following: Are disciplines unique? Do they articulate? Can one discipline reside within or overlap another? The final answer to these questions will provide important direction to the nature of shared scientific knowledge. That is, if disciplines fail to articulate, how is it possible to share knowledge? But if disciplines subsume other disciplines or have shared boundaries, who has definitive ownership and/or responsibility for the knowledge? Who makes decisions in the case of shared knowledge? How is society to have access to the knowledge?

Certain concepts in the philosophy still require further clarification. Although the generative philosophy of science has identified data, concepts, theories, and law as elements of the philosophy, no attempt has been made to delineate the specific nature of these concepts for nursing. What about concepts that relate solely to the role of the clinician, such as skills (e.g., bathing, temperature measurement)? What will constitute theory? Do current nursing models constitute theory? Can theory guide practice? For instance, will using Johnson's behavioral system model (see Grubbs, 1980) in practice change outcomes? Are theories that guide practice the only type appropriate for a practice discipline such as nursing? Should the goal of theory ever be to control behavior? Can theory from a practice discipline become a scientific law?

These questions present further challenges to and for the generative philosophy. Further, these questions challenge the discipline of nursing. During the 1960s, there was lively debate among nurses as to the appropriateness of theory and methods in nursing science, that is, nursing's philosophy of science. These discussions resulted in new direction and growth in the discipline. As the 1990s begin, further advances in nursing require reexamination of the foundations that became our beliefs about the nature of "true" science. It is anticipated that this philosophy can provide the impetus and focus for this reexamination. If nursing chooses not to examine its foundation, forward momentum may be stopped by these issues. But examination could mean a renewed momentum and clarification of nursing science. Even more important, clarification could provide society with a clearer understanding of the nature and contributions that can only come from nursing science.

Ultimately, the value of any philosophy of science lies in its ability to provide a broad scope capable of directing a variety of disciplines. This usefulness is determined not only by the disciplines but also by society. The generative philosophy of science reflects the beliefs, values, and goals of practice professions such as nursing, recognizing that professions are created by society to meet a societal goal or need. Use of the generative philosophy can facilitate the development and growth of practice disciplines by clarifying the disciplinary mission and giving credence to a variety of disciplinary members.

References

Allen, D. (1985). Nursing research and social control: Alternative modes of science that emphasize understanding and emancipation. *Image: Journal of Nursing Scholarship, 17*(2), 59-64.

Andreoli, K. G., & Thompson, C. E. (1977). The nature of science in nursing. *Image: Journal of Nursing Scholarship, 9,* 32-37.

Benner, P., & Wrubel, J. (1989). *The primacy of caring: Stress and coping in health and illness.* Menlo Park, CA: Addison-Wesley.

Bunting, S., & Campbell, J. C. (1990). Feminism and nursing: Historical perspectives. *Advances in Nursing Science, 12*(4), 11-24.

Carper, B. A. (1978). Fundamental patterns of knowing in nursing. *Advances in Nursing Science, 1*(1), 13-23.

Clarke, P. N., & Yaros, P. S. (1988). Research blenders: Commentary and response. *Nursing Science Quarterly, 1,* 147-151.

Donaldson, S. K., & Crowley, D. M. (1978). The discipline of nursing. *Nursing Outlook, 26,* 113-120.

Flaskerud, J., & Halloran, E. J. (1980). A framework for analysis and evaluation of conceptual models of nursing. *Nurse Educator, 5*(6), 10-14.

Gorenberg, B. (1983). The research tradition of nursing: An emerging issue. *Nursing Research, 32,* 347-349.

Gortner, S. R. (1983). The history and philosophy of nursing science and research. *Advances in Nursing Science, 5*(2), 1-8.

Grubbs, J. (1980). The Johnson behavioral systems model. In J. Riehl & C. Roy (Eds.), *Conceptual models for nursing practice.* New York: Appleton-Century-Crofts.

Hagell, E. I. (1989). Nursing knowledge: Women's knowledge. *Journal of Advanced Nursing, 14,* 226-233.

Jacox, A. K., & Webster, G. (1986). Competing theories of science. In L. H. Nicoll (Ed.), *Perspectives in nursing theory* (pp. 335-341). Boston: Little, Brown.

Keller, E. F. (1985). *Reflections on gender and science.* New Haven, CT: Yale University Press.

Kemeny, J. G. (1959). *A philosopher looks at science.* New York: Van Nostrand.

Kuhn, T. (1970). *The structure of scientific revolutions* (2nd ed.). Chicago: University of Chicago Press.

Kuhn, T. (1977). *The essential tension.* Chicago: University of Chicago Press.

Laudan, L. (1977). *Progress and its problems: Toward a theory of scientific growth.* Berkeley: University of California Press.

Masterman, M. (1970). The nature of paradigms. In I. Lakatos & A. Musgrave (Eds.), *Criticism and the growth of knowledge* (pp. 59-60). Cambridge: Cambridge University Press.

Munhall, P. L. (1982). Nursing philosophy and nursing research: In apposition or opposition? *Nursing Research, 31,* 176-177, 181.

Norbeck, J. S. (1987). In defense of empiricism. *Image: Journal of Nursing Scholarship, 19,* 28-30.

Phillips, J. R. (1988). Research blenders. *Nursing Science Quarterly, 1,* 4-5.

Popper, K. (1979). Science: Conjectures and refutations. In K. Popper, *Essays in philosophy of science* (pp. 176-191). Chicago: University of Chicago Press.

Ramos, M. C. (1987). Adopting an evolutionary lens: An optimistic approach to discovering strength in nursing. *Advances in Nursing Science, 10*(1), 19-26.

Reverby, S. (1984). *Ordered to care.* Boston: Allyn & Bacon.

Rogers, M. (1980). Nursing: A science of unitary man. In P. Riehl & C. Roy (Eds.), *Conceptual models for nursing practice* (2nd ed., pp. 329-337). New York: Appleton-Century-Crofts.

Silva, M. C., & Rothbart, D. (1984). An analysis of changing trends in philosophies of science on nursing theory development and testing. *Advances in Nursing Science, 6*(2), 1-13.

Thompson, J. (1985). Practical discourse in nursing: Going beyond empiricism and historicism. *Advances in Nursing Science, 7*(4), 59-71.

6

Science as Problem Solving

SARA T. FRY

The nature of nursing science has undergone several interpretations during nursing's short history. Traditional views of science such as empiricism or positivism (Hempel, 1966), rationalist schools of thought (Popper, 1962), and revolutionary views (Kuhn, 1970) greatly influenced the development of nursing science during the 1950s and 1960s. In recent years, however, new influences on the nature of nursing science are occurring from evolutionary views of science (Toulmin, 1972), feminist views (Harding, 1986), and pluralistic views (Rorty, 1979).

These influences are increasingly evident in the nursing literature. For example, the deconstruction of nursing science is advised to eradicate knowledge development activities from limiting "dogmas" (Rodgers, 1991), and evolutionary models of theory evaluation are encouraged for more cogent and optimistic assessments of theoretical progress within nursing (Ramos, 1987). More recently, alternative linkages between philosophy, theory, and method in nursing science have been encouraged to promote a pluralistic approach to nursing science (Kim, 1993), and multiple modes of inquiry and multiple types of knowledge and theory are advocated so that nursing science can more adequately address all aspects of human reality (Wolfer, 1993).

A common thread in contemporary views about the nature of nursing science is the notion that nursing science should solve problems that are considered important/significant by the members of the discipline. This expectation about nursing science should not surprise us. Nursing is a practice discipline. The purpose of nursing activity is to treat human responses to potential and actual health problems (American Nurses' Association, 1980). Hence it is reasonable to expect the science of nursing to provide reliable and valid approaches, techniques, and theory that will enable nurses to practice effectively while solving problems. For this reason, the work of philosopher of science Larry Laudan has been of great interest to nurse scientists in recent years.

Laudan's Approach to Scientific Progress

In his critique of Kuhn's (1970) account of scientific revolutions, Laudan (1984) exposes the major flaws of Kuhn's view of scientific change and states unequivocally that it is time to acknowledge that Kuhn's *Structure of Scientific Revolutions* is no longer a credible account of scientific change. This is the assumption behind Laudan's (1977) seminal work, *Progress and Its Problems.* Asserting that scientific change simply does not occur in a revolutionary manner, he offers another account of scientific progress—evolutionary change—calling it "a more satisfactory account" because it answers more questions for science than does Kuhn's account.

The pragmatic character of Laudan's account is evident in his statement of the aim of science. For him, science's aim is not to establish truth about the world as we know it but simply to solve problems. Thus theories are evaluated and accepted on the basis of their problem-solving effectiveness, taking into consideration the number and importance of the empirical problems solved by the theory, the number and importance of the anomalies still unanswered by the theory, and the number and importance of the conceptual problems generated by the theory.

Central to Laudan's account of scientific progress is a rejection of traditional conceptions of truth regarding scientific theories. Earlier views of scientific progress in the philosophy of science all included some notion of truth. Scientific progress was usually seen as a successive attainment of the truth by a process of approximation and self-correction. Theories were even judged in terms of whether or not they brought us closer to the truth about the world, had more explanatory power, or, in the Popperian sense, told us what was clearly false about the world.

Laudan (1977), however, stands this usual view of the nature of science "on its head" (p. 125). For him, rationality involves some judgment of what it is that increases the problem-solving effectiveness of theories that we accept. It is even possible to espouse a view of rationality that presupposes nothing about the veracity or verisimilitude of the theories judged to be rational or irrational. Truth about the world is not what is at issue. Thus Laudan proposes a view of scientific rationality that is both refreshing and exciting in terms of contemporary discussions on nursing theorizing and the philosophy of nursing science:

> Philosophers and scientists since the time of Parmenides and Plato have been seeking to justify science as a truth-seeking enterprise. Without exception, these efforts have foundered because no one has been able to demonstrate that a system like science, with the methods it has at its disposal, can be guaranteed to reach the "Truth," either in the short or in the long run. . . . Realizing this dilemma, some philosophers have sought to link scientific rationality and truth in a different way—by suggesting that although our present theories are neither true nor probable, they are closer approximations to the truth than their predecessors. However, even these accounts are flawed because . . . no one has been able even to say what it would mean to be "closer to the truth" let alone offer criteria for determining how we could assess such proximity. (pp. 125-126)

Laudan's point is that if scientific progress consists of a series of theories that represent an ever closer approximation to the truth, then science cannot be shown to be progressive. However, if one adopts the pragmatic maxim that (a) science is a system of inquiry for the solution of problems, (b) scientific progress consists in the solution of an increasing number of important problems, and (c) rationality consists in making choices that will maximize the progress of science, then we might be able to show to what extent science constitutes a rational and progressive system (Laudan, 1977).

Responding to the Skeptics' Questions

As a philosopher of science, Laudan recognizes that this view entails that scientists run the risk of adopting theories that are progressive and rational but are false. This situation, however, should not discourage the scientist. Many scientific theories in the past were proved false, and this will continue to happen in the future.

Does this mean that when this occurs we judge that science has not progressed? Certainly not, asserts Laudan (1977). Any theory of science will be worthy to the extent that it solves problems and contributes to scientific progress. He states, "The workability of the problem-solving model is its greatest virtue. In principle we can determine whether a given theory does or does not solve a particular problem" (p. 127).

How is the problem-solving effectiveness of a theory determined? Laudan assesses specific cases drawn from the history of the science. In nursing, this type of assessment might look like this: If we want to know whether or not to accept a specific theory to guide the practice of nursing, one evaluates all the applications of this theory to a specific set of problems in nursing care and evaluates how this theory has solved the problems. Next, one asks whether the application of the theory raised significant conceptual problems about the theory and left anomalous problems unanswered. One then evaluates how significant these conceptual problems are and whether the unanswered anomalous problems are significant ones for the discipline of nursing. Last, the answers to these questions are adjudicated against the number and significance of the solved problems from the application of the theory.

Laudan's account seems to offer nursing a way to evaluate scientific theory in terms of its problem-solving effectiveness in nursing practice. A particular theory could be evaluated by how well it solves problems in nursing practice that one typically brings theory to bear upon. The problem-solving effectiveness of the theory would be assessed in terms of the empirical problems solved, the conceptual problems generated by the theory, and the anomalous problems continued or left hanging. The process of theory evaluation is essentially a pragmatic calculus of problem-solving effectiveness.

What happens when scientists disagree about the significance of the solved problems? Laudan recognizes that agreement among scientists about the significance/nonsignificance of solved problems is not an easy task to achieve. He also recognizes that failure to agree can potentially affect

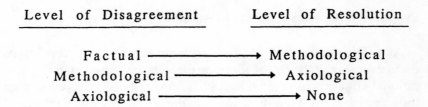

FIGURE 6.1. Hierarchical model of rational consensus formation
SOURCE: From Science and values: The aims of science and their role in scientific debate *(p. 27) by L. Laudan, 1984, Berkeley: University of California Press. Copyright 1984 by University of California Press. Reprinted by permission.*

the acceptability of theories as well as the reputation of the particular scientific community within the discipline. At issue in the agreement/ nonagreement debate is the role of cognitive values as a measure of the significance/nonsignificance of the solved problem.

Laudan (1984) explores the role of cognitive values in the shaping of our views about scientific rationality including the significance/ nonsignificance of the solved problem in *Science and Values.* He argues that *consensus* within a scientific discipline on the cognitive values that guide theory choice has not been easy to attain. Because of the difficult nature of this enterprise, Laudan bypasses the consensus issue and gives an account of *dissensus* instead. He argues that this approach will stimulate scientific theorizing and allow discussions of scientific rationality to proceed without presupposing a set of values that the scientists must agree on prior to beginning the discussion.

In explaining this approach in more detail, Laudan explores the usual way that philosophers of science have resolved disagreements about theory choice or achieved consensus on theory choice in the past. Assuming that disagreements in any science can exist at the factual, the methodological, or the axiological level (or the level of cognitive values), he asserts that disagreements at one level are usually resolved by appealing to another level (see Figure 6.1). For example, disputes over factual claims are usually resolved by appeals to methodology, and disputes over methodology are resolved by looking to the founding intentions or aims of the scientific community (the axiological level). When disputes occur at the axiological level, however, there is no way to resolve disagreements and reach consensus.

Kuhn (1970), of course, assumes this approach of resolving disagreements in his view of scientific change. When the members of the scientific community have disagreements at the axiological level, a "crisis" occurs that can only be resolved by a revolutionary change in the scientific discipline. Kuhn even cites examples from the history of science to support his view, which has had a powerful effect on how members of the scientific community have viewed the development of knowledge in their disciplines during the past 20 years.

Laudan, however, is very critical of this approach to consensus formation among members of the scientific community. He argues that scientists in a discipline can subscribe to different goals and that when this occurs it does not necessitate revolutionary change in the discipline for scientific progress to continue. Progress can be made in any discipline through continued research without recourse to a scientific revolution. For Laudan, scientific change can be rational *and* progressive while adjustments at the axiological level occur (or evolve) over time.

How does Laudan propose resolving disagreements about cognitive values? We must first change our thinking about disagreements over facts, methods, and the goals of science, he argues. Disagreements at all levels can and do exist within a discipline and among members of the scientific community at any given moment. For example, the science's phenomena of interest can be articulated differently or even be viewed differently by members of the discipline. Yet all inquiry about the phenomena can be considered fruitful and useful to the discipline, regardless of these differences. A similar view about the progress of nursing science has been argued in terms of avoiding closure on factual claims, methodologies, and even the phenomenon of interest within nursing science at the present time (Suppe, 1982).

Second, instead of a unidirectional model on consensus formation—from facts to method to aims—Laudan claims that we need a multidirectional model of scientific change. He proposes a "reticulated model" that allows for the use of knowledge gained from available methods of inquiry as a means to assess the viability of proposed cognitive aims or values (see Figure 6.2).

Laudan's model of scientific rationality allows for value formation and agreement on ideal goals even though there is no known method to achieve that value or goal of the scientific discipline. Likewise, value formation and agreement on ideal goals of the science can change whenever new information has been generated through the various methods

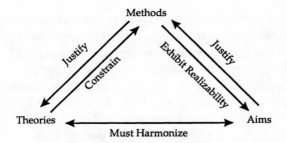

FIGURE 6.2. The reticulated model of scientific rationality
SOURCE: From Science and values: The aims of science and their role in scientific debate *(p. 63) by L. Laudan, 1984, Berkeley: University of California Press. Copyright 1984 by University of California Press. Reprinted by permission.*

of science. What actually occurs in the growth of a scientific discipline, Laudan claims, is a complex process of mutual adjustment and mutual justification among all levels of scientific commitment. Justification flows upward as well as downward in the hierarchy linking aims, methods, and factual claims in a dynamic manner. No one level of scientific achievement is considered more privileged than another, and mutual dependence exists between all three levels of inquiry. The model does not presuppose any single "right" goal for inquiry because Laudan considers it legitimate to engage in inquiry for a wide variety of reasons and purposes related to the discipline's phenomena of interest.

The Effect of Laudan's Model of Scientific Change on Theorizing

With this model of scientific change, it is easy to see that issues such as reaching agreement on the phenomena of interest or careful articulation of the disciplinary perspective are no longer important for scientific growth to occur. These issues are simply eclipsed so as to get on with the actual work of the scientific discipline. As Laudan (1984) states, "Those who imagine that there is a single axiology that can or should guide investigation into nature have failed to come to terms with the palpable diversity of the potential ends and uses of inquiry" (p. 64).

Diversity of inquiry even means that it is possible to include Kuhn's views about scientific change within the reticulated model of scientific rationality once the Kuhnian notion of paradigms is eliminated. In Kuhn's (1970) model, scientific paradigms have a particular view about the world. During a scientific revolution, whole paradigms are replaced or succeeded by competing paradigms that hold a different worldview. Laudan's (1984) model, however, allows for the replacement of component parts of a worldview when it is established that parts of the worldview do not encourage theorizing that solves problems. He states, "The problem of consensus is solved once we realize that the various components of a world view are individually negotiable and individually replaceable in a piecemeal fashion" (p. 73). There is simply no need for a wholesale replacement of theories or worldviews (paradigms or research traditions) by a scientific revolution once the evolutionary view of scientific change is accepted. What *is* necessary for scientific progress to occur is merely the elimination or replacement of those approaches that do not solve problems.

Laudan's views are clearly anchored within the thoughts of the early pragmatists, especially Peirce (1955) and Dewey (1960). The evaluation of theory is not made according to strict criteria that are determined prior to the valuative endeavor. Theory evaluation is centered on the problems solved by the theory. Assessment of scientific change involves moving back and forth between theories, methods employed to do science, and the aims of science. Each level of the process is justified by appealing to the other levels of the process. Scientific change is recognized when adjustments between the levels are required to accommodate changes in the central problems explored by the discipline, shifts in the basic explanatory hypotheses, and subtle changes in the rules of investigation employed by the discipline (Laudan, 1984).

Conclusion

The pragmatic approach exemplified by Laudan can be a powerful model for nursing science as the discipline becomes familiar with Laudan's work, his terminology, and his reticulated model of how science really works. Change is occurring in nursing science in an evolutionary manner, and the development of nursing knowledge is a reality. Scientific growth may be hard to see over a short period of time, but growth has certainly resulted from changes in the articulation and acceptance of the phenomena of nursing interest and can easily be observed by reading the nursing literature. Shifts in basic explanatory hypotheses related to nursing practice are also evident in nursing education, whereas changes in the unspoken rules about preferred methodologies to do nursing science are prominent in the nursing literature.

Laudan's approach to understanding these changes and scientific growth within the discipline should receive serious consideration by anyone interested in pursuing nursing's scientific identity during the last half of the 20th century.

References

American Nurses' Association, Congress for Nursing Practice. (1980). *Nursing: A social policy statement*. Kansas City, MO: Author.

Dewey, J. (1960). *The quest for certainty*. New York: Capricorn.

Harding, S. (1986). *The science question in feminism*. New York: Cornell University Press.

Hempel, C. G. (1966). *Philosophy of natural science*. Englewood Cliffs, NJ: Prentice Hall.

Kim, H. S. (1993). Identifying alternative linkages among philosophy, theory and method in nursing science. *Journal of Advanced Nursing, 18*, 793-800.

Kuhn, T. S. (1970). *The structure of scientific revolutions* (2nd ed.). Chicago: University of Chicago Press.

Laudan, L. (1977). *Progress and its problems*. Berkeley: University of California Press.

Laudan, L. (1984). *Science and values: The aims of science and their role in scientific debate*. Berkeley: University of California Press.

Peirce, C. S. (1955). *Philosophical writings of Peirce* (Selected and edited with an introduction by J. Buchler). New York: Dover.

Popper, K. R. (1962). *Conjectures and refutations*. New York: Basic Books.

Ramos, M. C. (1987). Adopting an evolutionary lens: An optimistic approach to discovering strength in nursing. *Advances in Nursing Science, 10*(1), 19-26.

Rodgers, B. L. (1991). Deconstructing the dogma in nursing knowledge and practice. *Image: Journal of Nursing Scholarship, 23*(3), 177-181.

Rorty, R. (1979). *Philosophy and the mirror of nature*. Princeton, NJ: Princeton University Press.

Suppe, F. (1982). Implications of recent developments in philosophy of science for nursing theory. In *Proceedings of the Fifth Biennial Eastern Conference on Nursing Research* (pp. 10-16). Baltimore: University of Maryland School of Nursing.

Toulmin, S. (1972). *Human understanding*. Princeton, NJ: Princeton University Press.

Wolfer, J. (1993). Aspects of "reality" and ways of knowing in nursing: In search of an integrating paradigm. *Image: Journal of Nursing Scholarship, 25*(2), 141-146.

An Evolutionary Approach to the Discipline of Nursing and Nursing Administration

CATHY RODGERS WARD

From the early part of the 20th century up to the 1960s the academic world of philosophy of science was dominated by formal methods of scientific inquiry and ideals, mathematical analysis, and conformity of scientific argument to permanent formal canons. During the 1960s, professional philosophers of science began to seriously study the historical development of science and confronted the historical, temporal world with its concrete detail, at the same time dismissing the formal abstractions of the previous generations (Toulmin, 1977). This shift in focus went from that of the "discipline oriented" researcher to that of the "problem oriented" researcher. Toulmin (1972) and Laudan (1977) formalized the problem orientation school of thought, which is referred to as "evolutionary." This chapter analyzes the influence of the evolutionary school of thought on the discipline of nursing, with an emphasis on the solving of conceptual problems, particularly in nursing administration. The process of conceptual change is discussed and includes examples of inward and outward understanding in nursing.

Background on the Evolutionary Model

AIMS OF SCIENCE

The evolutionary school of thought arose from the inability of previous approaches in the philosophy of science to adequately answer certain fundamental questions about the nature of scientific knowledge. For example, the question "What is the aim of science?" has been answered by the empiricists as moving toward the truth. The evolutionists refute this stance and declare that truth is not achievable and has no satisfactory semantic characterization (Laudan, 1981). From this perspective, the evolutionists also say that it is impossible for the logical positivists to answer the question of whether or not science progresses because it is impossible to know if one theory is truer than another. Evolutionists instead propose that the goals of science must be obtainable and their achievement verifiable.

Laudan (1977) suggests that the aim of science is to secure theories with a high problem-solving effectiveness. From this viewpoint, science progresses if successive theories solve more problems than their predecessors. Toulmin (1972) defines scientific problems as being the differences between a discipline's ability to explain salient features of the field and the explanatory ideals of those within the field. According to the evolutionists, the focus for scholarly activity of a discipline is the scientific problem.

THE NATURE OF PROBLEMS

There are two basic types of problems that coexist in science. Scientific progress is defined by the solution of these problems. These types of problems are referred to by Laudan (1977) as empirical and conceptual. Empirical problems are things about the natural world that strike us as odd or are otherwise in need of explanation. Traditionally, these problems are thought of as the "scientific" ones, and empiricists such as Popper (1968) believe that only empirical problems should govern choices of theories in science.

Conceptual problems are nonempirical and are characteristics of theories themselves. These problems represent a higher order of questions about science and about the structures designed to answer empirical questions. Conceptual problems allow for the combination of the questions "What is in fact the case about the world?" and "What are the explanatory empirical phenomena?" Asking these questions constructs a better representation of the aspects of Nature than asking either question alone would yield. Additionally, conceptual issues assist in determining more precisely on what conditions and with what degree of accuracy this representation of the aspects of Nature can be *applied* to explain the world.

THE EVOLUTIONISTS AND THE DISCIPLINE OF NURSING

The notion of conceptual or nonempirical issues having any relevance is antithetical to empiricists, certainly to many philosophies of science and exhibits a major leap in philosophic analysis. The evolutionists were the first to recognize the *application* of explanations and the social relevance of scientific inquiry and therefore promoted significant directional pathway changes in the philosophy of science. By acknowledging the importance of the application of scientific knowledge, the evolutionists opened the door for the discipline of nursing to be considered in the realm of the world of science. Often referred to as an "applied science," nursing's knowledge has need for application and also has definite social and political contextual ramifications. Two main themes in Toulmin's (1972) work are very relevant for nursing and will be further explored: a new definition of discipline and an examination of how conceptual change occurs within disciplines.

Toward a New Definition of Discipline

Toulmin (1972) poses several questions related to the definition of a discipline:

- At what point does intellectual activity have the character of a discipline?
- By what indexes should we determine that a discipline exists?
- What makes the later phases of a science the "legitimate heirs" of the earlier?

The answers to these questions are rooted in the idea of a continuing *genealogy of problems* (Toulmin, 1972), or problems that successive generations face. Nurses under Florence Nightingale's supervision faced problems such as nutrition and noise reduction for the sick. The former is a scientific problem for which many solutions have arisen in the past century. The latter problem of noise reduction in hospitals is just beginning to be systematically studied. Both problems remain concerns for nurses today, although progress on their solution varies.

Concerns can belong only to individuals; therefore, the question arises as to the role of individuals within a discipline. The idea that conceptual issues remain concerns of the people in a discipline over time supports Toulmin's premise that an intellectual discipline always involves both its concepts and the individuals who are concerned about them.

APPLICATION OF
KNOWLEDGE WITHIN A DISCIPLINE

A definition of a discipline by Toulmin (1972) allows for the application of knowledge generated by that discipline. There is room in a discipline for more than one type of knowledge, including theoretical (scientific knowledge) and praxis (technology and craft knowledge). Toulmin (1976) differentiates these two types of knowledge in the discipline of medicine as biomedicine (scientific knowledge) and general clinical medicine (praxis knowledge).

It follows that nursing can be described in a similar fashion whereby nursing's theoretical knowledge is that of "bionursing" or that gained from pursuing answers to empirical problems in nursing. Praxis knowledge in nursing is general clinical knowledge. While there is currently no such recognized terms as "bionursing," Toulmin (1976) points out that prior to World War II there was no such term as biomedicine and that medicine was not even remotely linked with science or scientific knowledge. The turn to science came as a result of technological developments in pharmacology and the availability of public funds to study the empirical problems of medicine. Similar parallels could be drawn in nursing over the past 20 years given the increased demand for rigorous research methods and the beginning of available public funds for researching nursing's empirical problems. The establishment of the National Institute for Nursing, which funds nursing research within the federal body of the National Institutes of Health, is an example of nursing's movement in the direction of pursuing scientific knowledge.

Toulmin (1976) would also recognize clinical knowledge in nursing as a type of knowledge (praxis knowledge) within a discipline and would include everything from the principles of nursing diagnosis and treatment to specific nursing diagnoses and treatments of specific patients. Ramos (1987), in reflecting on Toulmin's work, notes that problems in a discipline arise from the practice setting and that when practice changes, the discipline also changes. It is the concepts of the practice that reflect the state of knowledge in a discipline. Concepts in nursing change in response to environmental, social, or political factors.

Conceptual Change

Toulmin (1972) describes understanding as having both "outward looking" and "inward looking" activities. Outward-looking activities are those that look at mastering the problems posed by the world. Inward-looking activities of understanding are those that consider how it is that we master these problems. These descriptions are also appropriate for understanding in nursing. Outward-looking activities in nursing are those that master the problems of nursing practice and nursing science, whereas inward-looking activities are those that ask questions about the mastery of problems in nursing.

Individuals within the discipline may perform both activities, but those who are primarily interested in outward understanding may include practicing nurses, clinical nurse researchers, and "bionursing" scientists. Inward understanding in nursing tends to be pursued by nurse philosophers, nurse educators, nurse administrators, nurse historians, nurse ethicists, nurse attorneys, and nurse theorists. It is the inward-looking intellectual methods that paint the "epistemic self-portrait" of nursing. Pursuit of inward understanding in nursing involves seeking answers to the conceptual problems of the discipline.

INWARD UNDERSTANDING
AND NURSING ADMINISTRATION

One area of inward understanding within nursing is that of nursing administration. If science is a problem-solving and problem-oriented activity as proposed by the evolutionists, an argument can be made that the knowledge in nursing administration is scientific knowledge. Laudan (1977) describes problems as the focal point of scientific thought and theories as the end result. Nursing administrators have drawn on the theories of sociology, psychology, economics, education, and organizational development to solve problems confronting nursing administration. One example of this is the study of the phenomenon of staff satisfaction. This problem has been studied using motivational and other theories to the point where a body of knowledge now exists related to solving the problem of staff nurse job satisfaction.

The concept of nurse job satisfaction within the discipline is also evolving over time and is congruent with the evolutionist school of thought. For example, nursing administrators have previously been interested in nurse job satisfaction as it related to the problem of nurse turnover. More recently, the question of whether nurse job satisfaction actually impacts on patient outcomes has arisen as a problem of inquiry. Toulmin (1972) addressed in detail the notion of conceptual evolution as it relates to the evolutionist school of thought.

CONCEPTUAL CHANGE IN NURSING

Concepts frequently held as essential for the discipline of nursing are those of client, health, environment, and nurse. The first three concepts are essential in outward understanding, whereas the concept of nurse within the discipline of nursing is of interest for inward understanding. Inclusion of the study of nursing itself in the discipline confirms nursing as an intellectual discipline, according to Toulmin (1972), and allows for scholarly conceptual problem-solving activity to occur within the various segments of nursing including nursing administration.

Toulmin's (1972) model of evolutional conceptual change can be used to trace the evolution of concepts in nursing and can demonstrate the relationships between concepts of inward and outward understanding, including concepts in nursing administration and nursing practice (see Figure 7.1). This model depicts the genealogical development

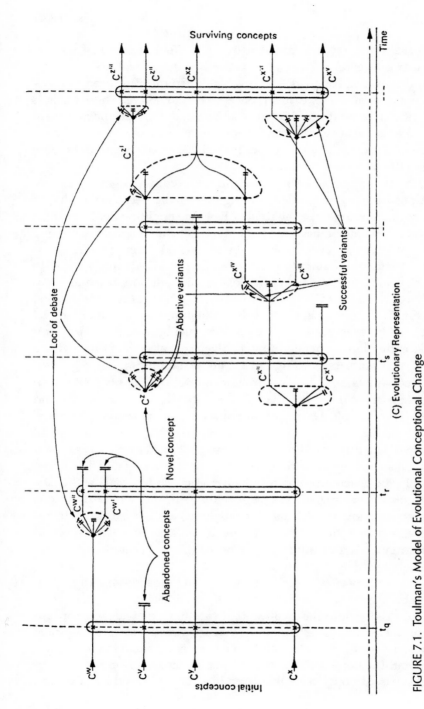

FIGURE 7.1. Toulman's Model of Evolutional Conceptional Change

SOURCE: Toulman, Stephen; Human understanding: The collective use & evolution concepts. Copyright © 1972 by Princeton University Press. Reprinted/reproduced by permission of Princeton University Press.

87

of relevant concepts in a discipline over time. Toulmin's model assumes that concepts enter the discipline rationally or for good reasons.

In this model, concepts may be abandoned or introduced as novel concepts and may vary to form conceptual innovations. These variants may either be considered aborted or successful by the discipline. Successful variants are surviving conceptual innovations over time. One example of a successful variant may be the evolution of primary nursing within the discipline of nursing.

Primary nursing arose in nursing from the concept of nurse-patient relationship (outward understanding), which has been an established concept in nursing since the time of Florence Nightingale. Over time, the strengthening of the nurse-patient relationship by primary nursing is accepted as a surviving concept in nursing. The conceptual innovation of primary nursing itself, however, has changed and "varied" to also develop innovations in care delivery models and, more recently, has been expanded to incorporate nurse-subordinate (nurse assistants) relationships, such as in Manthey's (1989) practice partnership model of care. In this example, a concept rooted in solving an empirical problem (seeking outward understanding) evolved into a concept for solving a conceptual problem (seeking inward understanding).

Successful variants of conceptual innovations will only continue in nursing if the conceptual change does not die with its creator and others in the discipline take up the innovation. The conceptual innovation of case management in nursing is another example of a successful variant of the concept of primary nursing. Whether or not case management survives as a successful innovation in nursing will depend on many factors, including the responsiveness of individuals within the discipline to take up the concept, development, and debate of the idea through professional forums of discussions, and, of course, external factors, such as reimbursement and health policy issues. Concepts that do not remain relevant for nursing or for nurses in the discipline are not likely to succeed over time.

Other concepts may be initiated into a discipline to solve an empirical problem or to seek knowledge about the clinical practice of nursing and then evolve into some conceptual variations that address conceptual problems and other variations that are directed toward empirical problems. Care of the transplantation patient is a concept that illustrates this point. The nursing care of transplant patients has given rise to many other areas of concern in the discipline, including ethical decision making and resource allocation by administrators and quality of life and immunosuppression by clinicians. This model would allow for this relationship of conceptual and empirical problems within a genealogical evolution of concepts.

There are some unanswered questions by Toulmin (1972) regarding conceptual change in a discipline. For example, Toulmin does not address whether evolutionary views can accommodate abandoned concepts that reoccur in a discipline. The reemergence of home care as a major setting for nursing care is a good example of this phenomenon in nursing (Brooks & Kleine-Kracht, 1983) as is the idea of bloodletting in the discipline of medicine. It is also not clear if there is a saturation point for viable concepts or if there are maximum or minimum numbers of concepts that are "ripe" at any given time in a discipline. Conceptual boundaries or areas of overlap with other disciplines are certainly discussed by Toulmin (1972) as being very possible, although the specific effects of these fluid boundaries are not discussed with respect to the model of evolutionary conceptual change.

Summary and Conclusions

Since the development of the evolutionary school of thought by philosophers of science in the 1960s, the notion of human understanding and progress in science has been looked upon differently when compared with traditional views of science. The use and application of problem solving as a focus of science and of intellectual disciplines has allowed for the discipline of nursing to be viewed as a scientific one. The writings of Florence Nightingale in the 1850s reflect a problem-solving approach to the science of nursing as she posed both empirical and conceptual problems. Recognizing the critical elements of both knowing and being aware that we are knowing beings, the evolutionary approach encompasses all the essential concepts of nursing.

Nursing administration can be considered a field of scientific inquiry within the evolutionists' framework as the body of knowledge within nursing administration is forming to solve problems of interest to the discipline. This evolutionist school of thought also reveals inward and outward understanding in a discipline, thus recognizing nursing administration as a valid area of scientific inquiry. Toulmin's (1972) model of conceptual change, in sharp contrast to previous philosophic analyses of concepts, can accommodate the complexity of nursing's problems as well as the evolution of concepts within the discipline of nursing over time. This dynamic approach to conceptual change promotes the evolution of nursing knowledge at varying speeds and is more reflective of the reality of the evolution of the discipline of nursing than are other traditional views.

References

Brooks, J. A., & Kleine-Kracht, A. E. (1983). Evolution of a definition of nursing. *Advances in Nursing Science, 5*(4), 51-63.

Laudan, L. (1977). *Progress and its problems: Towards a theory of growth.* Berkeley: University of California Press.

Laudan, L. (1981). A problem-solving approach to scientific progress. In I. Hacking (Ed.), *Scientific revolutions* (pp. 144-155). New York: Oxford University Press.

Manthey, M. (1989). Practice partnerships: The newest concept in care delivery. *Journal of Nursing Administration, 19*(2), 33-35.

Popper, K. (1968). *The logic of scientific discovery.* New York: Harper.

Ramos, M.C. (1987). Adopting an evolutionary lens: An optimistic approach to discovering strength in nursing. *Advances in Nursing Science, 10*(1), 19-26.

Toulmin, S. (1972). *Human understanding: The collective use and evolution of concepts.* Princeton, NJ: Princeton University Press.

Toulmin, S. (1976). On the nature of physicians' understanding. *Journal of Medicine and Philosophy, 1*(1), 32-50.

Toulmin, S. (1977). From form to function: Philosophy and history of science in the 1950s and now. *Daedalus, 106*(3), 143-163.

III

Postmodern Philosophy of Science

Postmodern philosophies of science have challenged most tenaciously the traditional philosophies of science. The term postmodern has been interpreted broadly here to include all of those philosophies that have resolutely contested the objectification of knowledge. As such, postmodernism includes such philosophies as phenomenology, hermeneutics, feminism, critical theory, and poststructuralism. Not surprising, each and every one of these philosophies of science would object to this classification, for if these schools of thought have one trait in common it is their objection to being classified with any other school of thought. Each of these philosophies views itself as unique. In many ways they are.

Feminism is the first of the postmodern philosophical schools of thought to be presented in this section. Three chapters are devoted to exploring feminist beliefs regarding science and scientific knowledge. These contributions contemplate the relationships between science, scientific knowledge, and oppression. First, Ruth Ginzberg explores the intersections between feminism, science, and nursing. Second, Sandra Harding's seminal work on the search for a feminist method is presented. In an "Afterword," she reviews the dialogue generated by her original work and comes to the conclusion that the only major change called for is that of the dynamic relationship between knowledge and the researcher. Finally, Gayle Page contributes an application chapter exploring how scientific knowledge can and has been affected by gender issues in the development of our knowledge about pain and how that knowledge has been limited by gender bias.

The second postmodern philosophical school of thought presented in this section is phenomenology. It has often been noted that phenomenology is a philosophy, an approach, and a research method. The one commonality throughout all its permutations is its emphasis on knowledge as available from the phenomenon in the subjective lived experience. Anna Omery and Carol Mack discuss the philosophy of phenomenology and describe how four different phenomenological thinkers, Husserl, Heidegger, Schutz, and Merleau-Ponty, have viewed any possibility and/or probability for phenomenology to provide the philosophical foundation for science and scientific knowledge. Marlene Cohen contributes an application chapter using phenomenology as a clinical research method to describe the experience of surgery.

While any discrete distinction between phenomenology and hermeneutics is always controversial, in this text hermeneutics is treated as a separate school of thought. Richard Steeves and David Kahn distinguish hermeneutic knowledge as the knowledge of the interpreted experience. Francelyn Reeder provides an application of hermeneutic knowledge by describing the hermeneutics of choice in the journey of caring.

Any discussion of knowledge development would be incomplete without critical theory's tenets on science. Hesook Kim and Inger Holter contend that praxis and communicative action are the basis for the scientific foundation of nursing practice in their review of critical theory. They also provide an application of critical theory by exploring how this philosophy provides the foundation for a "new" method of inquiry.

Poststructuralism is the final postmodern philosophical school of thought discussed in this text. Laura Cox Dzurec explores the distinctions between structuralist empiricist science and the philosophy of poststructuralism. She distinguishes poststructuralism that aims to illustrate where and how the political realities direct life experiences and, as a result, knowledge development. Dzurec also contributes an application chapter in which she explores how the knowledge of and about mental illness has been influenced by the realities of politics.

8

Feminism, Science, and Nursing

RUTH GINZBERG

The Questions

Feminism, science, and nursing converge at an important theoretical and practical intersection. New questions about the nature and scope of this intersection continue to emerge; more important, many of them lead to other questions at least as often as they do to answers. For these reasons, no taxonomy of the issues could ever be complete. My hope here is that we might begin to sort out some of the varied levels of issues, both in theory and in practice.

Questions Involving the Nature and Scope of Science

One cluster of issues at this intersection focuses around the nature, scope, practices, and methodologies of science. The best known struggles over these issues, at least in the history of Western science prior to the 20th century, occurred around the time of the 17th century—a time of dramatic social, political, philosophical, and epistemic upheaval in Europe. The collection of events that came to be known in the Western world as the Scientific Revolution brought about many of the terminologies, methodologies, commitments, and procedures that we recognize today as Western science. However, since the publication in the 1960s of Thomas Kuhn's revolutionary book, *The Structure of Scientific Revolutions*, a new area of science studies has blossomed. Known by various names and carried on by a number of communities of investigators under various headings, it encompasses what might be called generally the social studies of science.

This collection of research foci, which includes critical theory and the sociology of knowledge as well as many feminist critiques of science studies, is largely predicated on the idea that science itself consists of socially embedded practices, policies, conventions, agreements, and political struggles that are not entirely separable from the knowledge they produce. Credit for the development of this variety of critiques appropriately goes back to the Frankfurt School, including such scholars as Adorno, Benjamin, Horkheimer, Marcuse, and, more contemporarily, Habermas. Yet certainly not all such critiques are products of the Frankfurt School's brand of critical theory. Thomas Kuhn's work, for example, came out of a diametrically opposed research tradition, which is part of what rendered it compelling to so many philosophers and historians of science, including many who had previously ignored critiques generated by the Frankfurt School. Meanwhile, philosophers from other traditions as varied as American pragmatism to logical positivism were simultaneously arriving at similar conclusions during the second half of the 20th century: that the knowledge produced by the practice of science could not escape the fact that it was a part of, and not outside of, the social and political traditions, structures, and constraints within which its production occurred. As those social and political traditions were challenged, so was the knowledge, and indeed the methodologies, of the science practices carried on within them.

Not unrelated to this is a growing recognition on the part of Western theorists that modern Western science is not the only science the world has known. While certainly not every knowledge claim is a scientific one, Paul Feyerabend and others demonstrated that it is very, very difficult to specify without recourse to political explanations why one sort of knowledge claim—usually the sort made by white men working within Western science culture—counts as science, while another—usually made by some other demographically, ethnically, or geographically positioned group—does not.

At the same time that these theoretical developments were coming to the fore, Western medicine, for example, began looking toward traditions originating outside modern Western science, such as acupuncture and meditation, for answers to some of its most perplexing problems. Researchers such as Barbara Ehrenreich and Diedre English also argued convincingly, for example, that women convicted of practicing witchcraft in the Middle Ages actually may have been the real empirical scientists of their time. Those accused and convicted of witchcraft, they claim, actually were empiricists: Typically, they were the women healers of their communities at a time when most communities never encountered a physician trained in any of the European universities. These women healers studied and observed the medicinal properties of local herbs and plants and used them accordingly to help relieve the ills of their families and friends. This was at a time when university-trained physicians were prescribing prayer, incantation, bloodletting, leeches, and other such remedies. It is rather dubious whether formal university medical science actually "won" in the competition between competing theories (university physicians versus community witch-healers) because it actually was more "successful" in promoting health and eliminating disease. There is a good case to be made that the stories we have been told about the history of Western science are not quite what they claim to be. There are clear gaps where superstition apparently did "win" over empirical observation and where observably successful practices were discounted or ignored in favor of practices that produced less in terms of measurably successful results. More researchers began to suspect that science itself might not be quite what it was cracked up to be.

QUESTIONS INVOLVING
THE NATURE AND SCOPE OF FEMINISM

Another cluster of issues focuses around the nature, scope, practices, and methodologies of feminism. In the second half of the 20th century, Western feminisms also have emerged as major social, political, and intellectual forces. However, feminism is not monolithic. The various strands of feminism raise a variety of differing issues, some of which are and some of which are not adopted or pursued by others of the various feminist projects. Indeed, disagreements between various strands of feminism often have produced lively and sometimes bitter internal debates between feminists about what sorts of concerns, practices, methods, and commitments are and are not "feminist." Although this ought to be perceived as a healthy sign of the intellectual and political vigor of feminism, it is often represented by opponents of feminism as a reason to deride feminist scholars, activists, projects, and insights.

Some feminisms have chosen to focus on gaining equal rights and opportunities for women that the most privileged Western men already enjoy. These strands of feminism often have made great strides in securing legislation and court rulings granting women workers pay equity and access to better paying but traditionally male-held jobs as well as voting rights, equal property and inheritance rights, legal equality within a marriage to the status of their mates, and other such legislative and judicial remedies. Within the context of home and family, these feminists often have been the ones who first argued for equal participation of fathers in parenting and housework activities and in equal access for male and female children to sports and scouting types of activities.

In the United States, equal-rights-oriented feminism owes a great deal to the African American civil rights movements of the mid-20th century, from which a great many insights and strategies were gained. Unfortunately, despite this political and intellectual debt, many African American and Latina women in the United States have felt marginal to white women's work toward gender equality, in part because the citizens with whom white women strove to be equal, were in fact middle-class white men. Many women of color saw little benefit in fighting for equality with economically underprivileged men of color, who were themselves often subjected to discriminatory forces at least as severe as any gender discrimination against middle-class white women. When white women imagined gaining access to jobs and pay traditionally available only to white men, they saw themselves gaining access to positions of power and policy making. However, when women of color imagined themselves gaining access to jobs and pay traditionally available only to men of color, they still saw themselves occupying underpaid, menial, or subservient positions with little or no political or economic power. Thus many women of color have felt that equal rights feminisms have ignored their situations and needs.

Other strands of Western feminism in the second half of the 20th century did pay more attention to issues of race and class, but because these strands' concrete political advances were less dramatic, they often had less prominent coverage in the news media and therefore had less effect on shaping public perceptions of "feminism." But that is not entirely the case. For example, feminisms that found their roots in issues of class were responsible for bringing the Marxist notion of "consciousness raising" to feminism. The feminist consciousness-raising or C-R group became a major tool of feminist education during the 1960s and early 1970s in the United States. These groups were responsible for helping many women come to see, often for the first time, that a lot of the things that made their lives feel futile, painful, unhealthy, unfulfilled, depressing, anxiety laden, hopeless, or empty were the result of systematic barriers common to all women and not just the result of personal inadequacies of adjustment. These directions owe much intellectual and practical debt to Marxist theories of class consciousness. Perhaps because of Western culture's general suspicion of communism during those cold war times, any activity owing even the mildest tip of the hat to Karl Marx for its theory or method was regarded with an inordinate amount of suspicion. Even labor union membership suffered during the cold war.

Another early and thick strand of feminism yielded fertile ground for the development of various attempts to discover what women's culture, art, music, psychology, politics, science, sexuality, and other practices might look like if women were free to pursue them without regard for whether or not men would approve of the results. This strand of feminism became known as radical feminism because of its intent to return to women's roots; the term "radical" is the Latin term meaning "root." Unfortunately, detractors of various sorts of radicalism have been able to link the term radical with terms such as "crazed," "wild-eyed," or "dangerous" in much of public perception and media coverage. These unfortunate attempts to produce derogatory word associations in the public's mind have rendered it difficult not only for radical feminists but also for radicals within other political movements to get a fair hearing for their ideas.

Radical feminism nurtured the development of, although it was not necessarily directly responsible for, such diverse feminist projects as the Boston Women's Health Book Collective, rape crisis centers and battered women's shelters, lesbian separatism, much feminist literary theory, the music known as Women's Music, ecofeminism and feminist peace politics, feminist psychotherapies, and indeed some of the attempts to ascertain whether there is, or could be, such a thing as gynocentric science. What these projects have in common is an underlying thread suggesting that what women do or would do when not co-opted by the interests and projects of men is distinctive and worth doing regardless of whether or how much it is devalued by men. This rests on a claim that women and men are different in important respects and that their projects, interests, concerns, and commitments may well be different.

One can see immediately why it is that radical feminist agendas and liberal or equal-rights-based feminist agendas often have clashed with one another. Whereas radical feminists have wanted to acknowledge, explore, and often emphasize differences between women and men, liberal feminists have wanted to de-emphasize those differences in order to argue that women and men deserved the same economic, legal, and political opportunities. These same struggles between liberal and radical agendas have been occurring within African American, Native American, Jewish, lesbian and gay, and other ethnic and demographic communities as well; they are not unique to feminism.

Who Cares?

As if these issues were not enough, there is another set of questions not yet addressed here about what constitutes nursing. Because the rest of this volume concerns itself with this question in far more detail than could be summarized here, I shall not attempt to do that. However, I do want to explore the notion of "care" because it resonates both with much of nursing's history and with some important contemporary feminist ethical theories, theories of knowledge, and philosophy of science. Some recent feminist theory regarding "care" is problematic, and I wish to caution against adopting the more problematic of these notions as a point of intersection between feminism and nursing sciences.

Relatively uncontroverted, I think, is that most nurses see their work ultimately as that of providing patient care. Some may distinguish the nursing profession from doctors' work exactly along a perceived boundary between care and objective science. Indeed, some nurses feel that nursing may be the last bastion of actual care remaining in an increasingly impersonal or bureaucratic health "care" system. Here is where a problem arises. Some express concerns about trends toward scientific nursing, fearing that the caring component of the nursing profession will be lost if nursing, too, becomes scientific in its orientation. This perspective may at first appear to mesh well with feminist ethical literature and theory, such as Carol Gilligan's discovery of a "different voice" that is more subjective and oriented toward "care" as well as being associated with women more often than with men. However, in effect, this view applied unmodified to nursing merely solidifies the stereotypical association of doctors with maleness, science, and objectivity while tightening the association of nursing with femaleness, nurturing, and subjectivity. The worry here is that this merely restates traditional gender role stereotypes and does little to theorize feminist change. In fact, it might even constitute a step backward rather than a step forward on some feminist measures of progress.

Recently, "care" itself has become a problematic notion within feminist philosophical literature. Since Gilligan's work in moral development theory that led to the publication of *In a Different Voice* in 1982, her so-called care ethic has been one of the most widely discussed issues in feminist theory. Gilligan's research findings contrasted a care ethic, which she found articulated most often by girls and women, with a so-called justice ethic, which she found articulated most often by boys and men. The justice ethic, she said, is the one described in most of the standard Western literature of philosophy, psychology, law, ethics, and child development theory. It focuses on fairness, impartiality, and reason as components of mature moral decision making. Little wonder that it should so dominate the standard Western literature, she claimed. Those works had been written almost entirely by men who thought they were speaking in a universal voice: a voice they believed spoke for and about everyone. But Gilligan heard another, different voice in women's narratives about moral decision making (hence the book's title). It was a voice of care, subjectivity, interpersonal connection, and particularity rather than a voice of impartiality, distance, and objectivity. This voice, she claimed, was largely, though not exclusively, the voice of women and girls. It was also largely absent from social, political, psychological, developmental, and philosophical theorizing that claimed to be about all humans. Perhaps worse, when it was not absent from such theorizing, it was characterized as a less mature stage of development along the way to "true" adult morality. This had the effect of continually casting the moral voices of women and girls as being, on average, less mature and less well developed than what was supposed to be everyone's gender-neutral ideal of "true moral maturity." Unfortunately, Gilligan said, this so-called true moral maturity was, at best, only one form of moral maturity: the form most often seen in middle-class white European and North American boys and men. Applying this standard to everyone left most others seeming, on the whole, less morally developed and more "primitive," a result she proceeded to challenge.

Finally, this sort of work has had a significant impact on feminist theories of knowledge and feminist conceptions of philosophy of science. One of the first to incorporate questions about women's distinctive voice into questions about science and knowledge was Evelyn Fox Keller, herself a molecular biologist, who was later to become the winner of a coveted McArthur Foundation "genius" award. Her biography of Barbara McClintock raised many of the basic questions about "women's subjectivity" and science.

Barbara McClintock is a Nobel prize recipient in biology, whose life and work in corn genetics was documented by Keller in her 1983 biography entitled *A Feeling for the Organism,* in which she presented McClintock as a scientist whose work was consistently unrecognized and underappreciated during most of her career. This much is an unfortunate but well-documented and uncontested fact. However, Keller's explanation was what was unusual. She relied on the feminist psychoanalytic work of early feminist philosophers of science to argue that McClintock's work was devalued as science just because of her observational stance: a personal connection, resembling that of care or concern, with the organisms with which she worked (the basis for the biography's title). Important here was Keller's assertion that science, indeed good science, indeed Nobel prizewinning science, could be, and sometimes is, conducted from a different perspective than that of the cool objective detachment that so many claim to be a necessary scientific stance. Going further, Keller claimed that this connected and caring perspective might well be the scientific parallel to Gilligan's "different voice" in moral development theory.

Who Knows?

When questions and goals regarding equality of opportunities are the defining questions and goals of feminism, that is, within the framework of liberal feminism, there is little need for controversy over the relationship between feminism and science. Liberal feminist goals have been primarily social and political goals, and where applicable, they applied to science as well as nonscience fairly unproblematically. For example, equal access to educational opportunities was presumed to mean equal access to science education as well as equal access to music education for both men and women. Demands, for example, that women be admitted to Ivy League schools included within their scope demands for access to Ivy League science educations as well as to Ivy League educations in history, government, fine arts, or any other disciplines of instruction. Demands for equal pay for equal work included demands for equal pay for scientists as well as equal pay for maintenance personnel. No special problems associated with science were encountered from within liberal feminist agendas per se.

They did emerge from radical and Marxist approaches to feminism, however. Suppose that preoccupation with objectivity turns out to be a particular feature of modern Western male psychology? This is, in fact, what many psychoanalytic and object relations theorists, including Nancy Chodorow, Dorothy Dinnerstein, Carol Gilligan, and Evelyn Fox Keller, argued early on. If that were true, would that make science's preoccupation with objectivity a particular feature of the demographics of those who defined it at the time of the Scientific Revolution (relatively privileged white christian European men)? Suppose women —defining themselves and their projects and concerns without reference to men—had also participated in the creation of Enlightenment science? Would it have turned out to have the same foci? Would there even have been a European Enlightenment as we now think of it, let alone science as we now know it? These questions left many feminists increasingly skeptical about any feminist project that merely injected women's increased participation into already defined conceptions and frameworks of science.

Some critics worry that "scientist" is an occupation, whereas "feminist" is a personal identity. The claim is that there is neither any particular tension between feminism and science, nor is there any particular resonance. They are simply thought to be independent variables.

Indeed, they are thought to be from wholly different spheres of one's life: One is from the personal or private sphere of individually held belief, and the other is from the public sphere of work, occupation, or professional engagement. The only possible points of conflict are thought to occur over the morality of certain experiments, projects, or procedures. (Does it violate my religious beliefs to perform tubal ligations? Is it against my moral principles to patch up injured soldiers just to send them back to the battlefront to be wounded again or possibly killed?) But these qualms are about the applications of scientific knowledge, not about the science itself, some might say. According to this view, although the uses to which scientific knowledge get put certainly are appropriate subjects for public debate, they are wholly separate from the science that produces the knowledge in the first place. The science that produces the knowledge itself is said not to be open to public debate or political criticism because its goal is the investigation of the natural world whatever that may be, not simply the investigation of some politically correct subset of the natural world. Enlightenment theories about what constitutes science claim that science is the process of "reading" the "Book of Nature." Human scientists are neither to write nor to censor what is found in that book; they merely are to read carefully and report accurately what they have learned.

Although it is beyond the scope of either this chapter or this volume to explore fully the claims of mid-20th-century feminist activists, one such claim, a famous one that many people have heard at one point or another, encompasses one of the earliest insights gained from feminist consciousness-raising groups of the 1960s: the claim that the personal is political.

This claim questions the division of the world into two different "spheres:" the personal, or private, sphere and the political, or public, sphere. The central point is that these two different spheres do not represent some sort of taxonomy of natural kinds. That is, there is no justification that precedes all political theorization for presuming that these two different spheres actually exist, aside from their creation by political theorists. The criticism is that the designation of some human activities as "personal" or "private" while others are designated "political" or "public" is itself a political theory and one that may not be neutral with respect to the distribution of its benefits. In particular, more than one feminist has noticed that those human activities designated personal or private most often have been assigned to women:

activities involving home, hearth, care and nurturing of the young, awareness of and attention to human emotions, attention to cleanliness and removal of evidence of dirt and decay, preparation and service of food, attention to the individual needs of those who are giving birth or dying, and maintenance of "family ties." Meanwhile, those human activities designated "political" or "public" most often are assigned to men: government, war, creation and explication of laws, development of theory, recording of history, construction of the permanent artifacts of civilization, formal education beyond childhood, and the reading of the "Book of Nature" (science). Concomitantly, those activities traditionally assigned to the private sphere typically also have been assigned relatively less value and relatively less importance than those activities traditionally assigned to the public sphere. Evidence of this unequal valuation is readily available in the historically low wages paid to those who perform work traditionally assigned to the private sphere, including child-care providers, cleaning personnel, food service workers, teachers of children, and, of course, nurses.

There are several possible remedies to this problem. One is to demand more equitable revaluation of various talents and skills while leaving the categories of "public" and "private" more or less unquestioned. This is the approach often taken by labor unions, for example, in striving to achieve wage equity between job categories that traditionally have been "female" and those that traditionally have been "male." For example, work skills may be divided according to degrees of difficulty and educational levels required for their performance. Often, numerical scores are assigned for various degrees of difficulty and educational levels of attainment under such a schema. This may be a practical solution for the late-20th-century workplace, but it is not one that challenges the underlying, and often unarticulated, theory behind these wage equity difficulties. Another possible approach, which is more relevant to the question of nursing's relation to both feminism and science, is to question the division of the life-world into categories of "public" and "private."

"Whose interests does it serve," one might ask, for example, "to continue to hold that what goes on between children, or severely disabled, or very elderly members of the community, and the people who care for them, belongs in the 'private' rather than the 'public' realm?" This sort of question prods not only at the very seams of the public/private split but also at the division of responsibility for those realms or spheres into male and female gender assignments. It also questions the easy assignments of science and politics to the public realm while care for the young, the sick, the disabled and wounded, and the very old remain assigned to the private sphere. It also provides the beginnings of a challenge to the separation of theory and practice. Historically, those most involved in doing the hands-on care in daily life have had little time to engage in politics or science or the construction of theories about their own work. But if there were no division between public and private, wouldn't the gulf between theory and practice, especially in fields such as nursing, begin to fall away as well?

Let us pause momentarily to dispel a common misconception about retheorizing the public/private split: Doing away with the theoretical split between "public" and "private" spheres does not entail or propose bringing sexual, excretory, or other "bedroom" or "bathroom" functions into the streets, shopping malls, or other "public spaces" of America any more than Marxist political theory suggests taking away people's individual toothbrushes and turning them into government property (which it does not, but which is another, similar, misconception).

What it would do, however, is take away the convenient wall that places "feminist" in the category of private belief and "scientist" in the category of public occupation. Rather than merely mixing apples and cucumbers, it would, indeed, upset the produce bin entirely. The hope, to continue this metaphor perhaps just a tad further than it deserves, is that this would produce new and healthful combinations that would be better for us in the long run than the old "theoretical salads" they replace, whose histories come from times and places no longer reflective of our current lives and social needs here and now.

Who's Asking?

At the close of the 20th century, many people, some of whom have been at least in part inspired by feminist theorists, are beginning to ask different kinds of questions about the theory and practice of science. A large number of knowledge theorists have given up on the notion of wholly objective pieces of truth, which merely sit around in the universe waiting to be discovered, like unclaimed gems embedded in an otherwise useless stone.

Now we wonder things like what is the role of context in the production or acceptance of knowledge claims? What is the role of the observer? What is the role of culture(s)? How much influence does the social construction of both observers or scientists, and observations or data, have on the activities of knowledge production? How much influence do those things have on the formulation of the questions which science practitioners will pose to the natural world? Is it desirable or necessary for the "knowing" (epistemic) Self and the moral Self to be one and the same Self within any given person?

These sorts of questions may seem abstract or remote and unconnected with the theory or practice of nursing, but in concrete ways they already affect many aspects of nursing research, practice, and theory. Undoubtedly, they will continue to do so. Lorraine Code, for example, has already applied an explicitly feminist epistemology (theory of knowledge) to her analysis of knowledge claims made by health care providers in a notorious Canadian court case. Analyzing transcripts and other court documents, she asks questions such as why is it that doctors were asked to testify about what they "knew" about patients while nurses were asked to testify about their "experiences" with those same patients? What is involved in the production and interpretation of knowledge claims, such that doctors were presumed to be involved in generating "knowledge" about patients while nurses were only presumed to be generating "experience"? What is the relation of "knowledge" claims to claims of "experience"? What does that have to do with gender relations? Power relations? Expectations about who is capable of knowing? Why is this the case? Should it be? What, if anything, needs our theoretical, philosophical, or political attention in response to such presumptions?" Questions such as these and others that emerge from the intersection of feminism and science studies will undoubtedly affect the theory and practice of nursing throughout the lifetimes of nurses currently working in, or preparing to work in, the field.

References

Code, L. (1991). *What can she know? Feminist theory and the construction of knowledge*. Ithaca, NY: Cornell University Press.

Gilligan, C. (1982). *In a different voice*. Cambridge, MA: Harvard University Press.

Keller, E. F. (1983). *A feeling for the oganism: The life and work of Barbara McClintock*. New York: Freeman.

9

The Method Question

SANDRA HARDING

Over the last two decades the moral and political insights of the women's movement have inspired social scientists and biologists to raise critical questions about the ways that traditional researchers have explained gender, sex, and relations within and between the social and natural worlds. From the beginning, criticisms of traditional research methods have generated speculations about alternative feminist methods. Is there a feminist method of research that can be used as a criterion to judge the adequacy of research designs, procedures and results? Is there a distinctive method that should be taught to students wanting to engage in feminist inquiry? If so, what is it?

My point in this chapter is to argue against the idea of a distinctive feminist method of research. I do so on the grounds that preoccupations with method mystifies what have been the most interesting aspects of feminist research processes. Moreover, I think that it is really

NOTE: © by Sandra Harding. Reprinted from Hypatia, vol. 2, no. 3 (Fall, 1987) with permission of the author and the publisher.

a different concern that motivates and is expressed through most formulations of the method question: What is it that makes some of the most influential feminist-inspired biological and social science research of recent years so powerful? I begin by indicating some variants of the method question and their diverse origins.[1]

Origins of Questions About Methods

We can now see that many androcentric assumptions and claims have survived through the years within, but unquestioned by most researchers in, traditional areas of biology and the social sciences.[2] In pondering the sources of such partial and distorted accounts, feminists have criticized the favored methods of their disciplines. They argue that prescription of only a narrow range of methods has made it impossible to understand women's "natures" and lives or how gender activities and commitments influence behaviors and beliefs. For instance, it is a problem that most social scientists have not questioned the practice—indeed, have sometimes overtly prescribed it—of having only men interview only men about both men's and women's beliefs and behaviors. It is a problem that biologists prescribe that cosmetics be tested only on male rats on the grounds that the estrus cycle unduly complicates experiments on female rats. It is a problem that Lawrence Kohlberg did not wonder about why he was finding women's responses to his moral dilemmas less easy than the men's responses to sort into the categories he had set up. As Gilligan (1982) pointed out, Kohlberg thereby replicated the assumption of Freud, Piaget, and Ericson that the patterns of moral development characteristic of men should be regarded as the model of human moral development. Faulty methods of inquiry appear to be implicated in these and many other such cases.

Moreover, it is not just particular research methods that are the target of feminist criticisms but the fetishization of method itself. The practice in every field of choosing research projects because they can be completed with favored methods amounts to a kind of methodolatry (in Mary Daly's memorable phrase) that sacrifices scientific explanation and increased understanding to scientistic fashions in research design (Daly, 1973, p. 11). For example, Sherif's (1979) survey of changing fashions in methods during the past half-century of psychology documents how this field attempted to gain legitimacy through blind imitation of what it wrongly took to be scientific methods. In imitating only the style of natural science research, psychology has produced distorted images of its subject matters. Historians of science join Sherif in arguing that the attempt to legitimate a new field in inquiry by claiming that it uses scientific method even more rigorously than its predecessors frequently masks scientisms of the flimsiest sort (e.g., Fee, 1980).

Responding to these criticisms of mainstream methods, a number of proposals for alternative feminist methods have emerged; I mention three that are well known. MacKinnon (1982) has argued that "consciousness-raising is feminist method" (p. 519). (She does so in the course of important criticisms of attempts to fit feminist analyses of rape and other acts of violence against women within the constraints of liberal and Marxist legal theory.) Even though this claim captures an intuitively important truth about feminist thought, it leaves biologists and social scientists puzzled about what, exactly, they should do differently in their laboratories, offices, or fieldwork. MacKinnon is thinking of method in ways very different from uses of the term in "methods" courses in the social sciences or in lab work in biology. Although this is certainly not a good reason to reject or ignore MacKinnon's point, it does motivate a closer examination of just what role unique methods play in feminist inquiry.

Hartsock (1983) argues for a "specifically feminist historical materialism." By replicating in the title of her chapter components of the method of Marxist political economy ("dialectical historical materialism"), she appears to hold that it is a method of inquiry as well as an epistemology she is explicating. Other social scientists have also pointed to the benefits of adapting Marxist method to the needs of feminist inquiry (Hartmann, 1981). Are methodology and epistemology also at issue in such discussions of method? It would be reasonable to argue that these analyses provide methodologies for feminism, not methods for feminist inquiry. That is, they show how to adapt the general structure of Marxist theory to a kind of subject matter that Marxist political economy never could fully appreciate or conceptualize. Is it method, methodology, theory, or epistemology that is the issue here? Is there any point to trying to distinguish these in such cases?

A third candidate for the feminist method arises from sociologists who favor phenomenological approaches. They appear to argue that feminist method is whatever is the opposite of excessive empiricism or of positivist strains in social research. In particular, they focus on

the virtues of qualitative versus quantitative studies and on the importance of the researcher identifying with rather than objectifying her
(women) subjects (e.g., Stanley & Wise, 1983). These critics draw attention to misogynistic practices and scientistic fetishes in social inquiry
that frequently have had horrifying consequences for both theory and
public policy. However, the prescription of a phenomenological approach as *the* feminist method ignores many of the well-known problems
with such ways of conducting social research. (These are problems also
for approaches to social inquiry labeled intentionalist, humanistic, or
hermeneutical.) For example, there are things we want to know about
large social processes—how institutions come into existence, change
over time, and eventually die out—that are not visible through the lens
of the consciousnesses of those historical actors whose beliefs and
activities constitute such processes. Moreover, the subjects of social inquiry are often not aware even of the local forces that tend to shape
their beliefs and behaviors, as Freud, for instance, pointed out. The
explanation of "irrational" beliefs and behaviors is just part of this
subject matter that is not amenable to phenomenological inquiry processes alone. Furthermore, these approaches do not fully appreciate
the importance of critical studies of masculinity and men (in the
military, the economy, the family, etc.) nor of feminist critical studies
of women's—including feminists'—beliefs and behaviors. Finally, what
would it mean for biology to use these approaches? Or, is feminism to
insist anew on just the division between nature and culture it has been
so successful in problematizing?

A different source of debate over method arises from the fact that
men and women social scientists who want to begin to contribute to
the feminist research agendas sometimes express puzzlement about
whether there is a special method that must be learned to do feminist
research. If so, what is it? Their disciplinary literatures are peppered
with references to "empirical method," "phenomenological method,"
and sometimes even "Marxist method," so it seems reasonable to seek
the feminist method. Such a method obviously should be included as
one of the alternative research methods taught in every social science.

No doubt some of these researchers are also perplexed about how
to conceptualize alternatives to the very common, although (they are
willing to grant) sexist practices of their disciplines because they have
been taught to think about methods of inquiry as the general categories
of concrete research practices. As one sociologist protested, there are

only three methods of social research: listening to what people say (in response to questions or in spontaneous speech), observing what they do (in laboratory situations or in the field, collectively or individually), and historical inquiry. Therefore, she argued, there cannot be a feminist method of inquiry. Yet she would admit that the problem of eliminating androcentric results of research appears to require more than simply having well-intentioned individuals conduct research because we know that individual intent is never sufficient to maximize objective inquiry. After all, where is the feminist inquirer who has not come to understand the inadequacy of some of her or his own earlier practices and beliefs? What are the implications of feminist critiques and counterproposals for conceptions of method such as this common one?

Finally, it is the use of a particular method of inquiry—scientific method—that is supposed to make the results of Galileo's and Newton's research so much more valuable than those of the medieval theologians whose accounts of astronomy and physics modern science dislodged. If feminist researchers are criticizing scientific method, it appears to some that they must be proposing some *nonscientific* method of inquiry. Although this train of thought usually emerges from critics hostile to feminism, at least traces of it appear in the thinking of some feminists. The latter are outraged—and properly so—at the distortions and subsequent policy crimes committed in the name of science, but they cannot see how to reform or transform science so as to eliminate those consequences that are so damaging to women. Accepting scientists' frequent claim that the true foundations of science are to be found in its distinctive method, they claim that science and its method are part of the problem against which feminism must struggle.

These discussions, meditations, claims, and analyses create a rich and confusing field for thinking about method. I turn next to some traditional distinctions between methods, methodologies, and epistemologies—and to some traditional confusions about some of these.

Method Versus Methodology Versus Epistemology

Philosophers have favored a distinction between method and methodology.[3] Will this distinction help us to sort out what is at issue in the method question?

METHOD

A research *method* is a technique for gathering evidence. Thus the feminist sociologist's focus on listening to what subjects say, observing them, or searching through historical records names categories of concrete techniques for gathering evidence. How unique to feminism are the techniques of evidence gathering used in the most widely acclaimed examples of feminist research? Is it to these techniques that we can attribute the great fecundity and power of feminist research in biology and the social sciences? Gilligan (1982) listens to what women say when presented with familiar examples of moral dilemmas—a traditional method of inquiry, according to the sociologist cited earlier—but uses what she hears to construct a powerful challenge to the models of moral development favored by Western psychologists (and philosophers). Sociologists observe men's and women's uses of public spaces—a traditional way of gathering evidence—but conclude that suburbs, usually thought of as desirable worlds for women, are in fact hostile to women's needs and desires (Werkerle, 1980). Kelly-Gadol (1976) examines ancient property and marriage records—yet another traditional research method—and goes on to argue that women did not have a renaissance, at least not during the Renaissance. The progress of (some) men appears to require loss of status for all women at those moments Western cultures evaluate as progressive.

Obviously, some of the most influential feminist researchers have used some very traditional methods. Of course, they do begin their research projects by listening more skeptically to what men say and more sympathetically to what women say; they observe both men and women with new critical awarenesses; they ask different questions of history. I will explore further how best to characterize these kinds of differences between feminist and traditional research. However, at this point it is reasonable to conclude that, in a way of characterizing research methods that is common in the social sciences, it is traditional methods that these feminist researchers have used.

This line of argument at least has the virtue of making feminist research appear acceptable as social science to those who had doubts. After all, it is using familiar methods of research: What more could one ask? However, this benefit is sometimes inadvertently bought at the cost of providing support for continued willful ignorance about feminist research on the part of such skeptics. If there is a way of arguing that there is "nothing new here," such critics can say to themselves and to others, "why read it, teach it, be concerned with it at all?" As a political strategy, there are both benefits and risks to the way of thinking about feminist research methods that I have been proposing.

Androcentric critics are not the only audience for answers to the method question, and they will, no doubt, rarely run out of self-convincing reasons to continue in their ways. Feminists, too, have claimed to identify a distinctive method in feminist research processes, and it would be a service to our own discourses if we could gain greater clarity about whether we should be making such claims. Can we conclude at this point that there is both less and more going on in feminist inquiry than new methods of research? The "less" is that it is hard to see how to characterize what is new about these ways of gathering evidence in terms of methods. The "more" is that it is new methodologies, epistemologies, and other kinds of theories that are requiring new research processes.

METHODOLOGY

Traditional philosophers have contrasted methods with methodologies. A *methodology* is a theory and analysis of "the special ways in which the general structure of theory finds its application in particular scientific disciplines" (Caws, 1967, p. 339). Here is surely one major place we should look to discover what is distinctive about feminist research. At least since Kuhn (1970) it has been clear that methods of inquiry cannot be regarded as independent of the general theories, specific hypotheses, and other background assumptions that guide research (e.g., optical assumptions guiding inferences from observations; logical assumptions about the appropriate structure of inferences; assumptions about computers, questionnaires, and other scientific "instruments"; assumptions about the veracity of historical archives) (Harding, 1976). Surely, it is the great innovations in feminist theory that have led to gathering evidence in different ways—even if this evidence gathering still falls into such broad categories as listening to what people say, observing them, and historical inquiry. For example, discussions of how sociobiology or psychoanalytic theory or Marxist political economy or phenomenology should be used to understand various aspects of women and gender addressed by different disciplines are methodology discussions that lead to distinctive research agendas—including ways of gathering evidence. Feminist researchers have argued that these theories have been applied in ways that make it difficult to understand women's participation in social life or to understand men's activities as gendered (versus as representing "the human"). They have transformed these theories to make them useful in such neglected projects.

The traditional definition of methodology with which I began here makes it appear that all theoretical discussions should be subsumed under the heading "methodology." But isn't a discussion about how to apply Marxist categories to analyses of women's role in reproduction different from a later discussion that assumes the results of the earlier one and goes on to hypothesize what that role is? Clearly, the choice of a substantive feminist theory of any kind will have consequences for what can be perceived as appropriate research methods. Do excessively empiricist (positivist) antitheoretical tendencies in the social sciences make some feminist researchers find it more comfortable to talk about competing "methodologies" rather than about competing theories? Should the fundamental distinctions here be between methods, substantive theories (and "methodology" discussions will help select these), and epistemologies? Not a great deal turns on answers to these questions—I certainly do not wish to replicate traditional philosophical fetishization of distinctions—but asking such questions heightens awareness of the extent to which our thinking is still constrained by distorting remnants of positivism.

EPISTEMOLOGY

It might be assumed that for a philosophical audience little needs to be said about what an *epistemology* is. It is, of course, a theory of knowledge, "concerned with the nature and scope of knowledge, its presuppositions and basis, and the general reliability of claims to knowledge" (Hamlyn, 1967, pp. 8-9). However, the fact that everyone could agree to this definition masks some important conflicts between feminist epistemological activity and traditional ways of thinking about the subject. For one thing, the mainstream Anglo-American tradition has sharply distinguished epistemology from philosophy of science. The former is construed as analyses of the nature and scope of "ordinary" knowledge. The latter is construed as analyses of the nature and scope of explanation for the natural sciences in general and/or for particular sciences. Insistence on this rigid distinction shields both fields from the kinds of epistemological questions arising from feminist scientific research. It makes it difficult to recognize those questions as either epistemological or as ones in the philosophy of science because they openly link the two domains. (Of course, it is also a problem for many traditional thinkers that these questions arise from social science and biology, not from physics or astronomy, and that they are feminist.) Such thinkers forget how the contours of modern epistemology have been designed and redesigned in response to the thought of Copernicus, Galileo, Newton, and later natural and social scientists.

Feminist epistemologies are responses to at least three problems arising from research in biology and the social sciences. First, if scientific method is such a powerful way of eliminating social biases from the results of research, as its defenders argue, how come it has left undetected so much sexist and androcentric bias? Is scientific method impotent to detect the presence of certain kinds of widespread social bias in the processes and results of inquiry? Second, is the idea of woman as knower a contradiction in terms? The issue here is not the existence of individual women physicists, chemists, astronomers, engineers, biologists, sociologists, economists, psychologists, historians, anthropologists, and others. There have been many of these throughout the history of science, and they have made important contributions to this history (Alic, 1986; Rossiter, 1982). Instead, the issue is that knowledge is supposed to be based on experience, but male dominance has simultaneously insured that women's experience will be different from men's and that it will not count as fruitful grounds from which to generate scientific problematics or evidence against which to test scientific hypotheses. Feminist research in biology and the social sciences has "discovered" and made good use of this lost grounds for knowledge claims, but the idea that more objective results of research can be gained by grounding research in distinctively gendered experience is a problem for traditional thinking in epistemology and the philosophy of science—to understate the issue. Finally, the more objective, less false, and so forth results of feminist research clearly have been produced by research processes guided by the politics of the women's movement. How can the infusion of politics into scientific inquiry improve the empirical quality of the results of this research? ("Think of Lysenkoism! Think of Nazi science!")

These kinds of questions about knowers and knowledge appear to be ruled out of court by this popular Anglo-American philosophical definition of what is to count as epistemology and as philosophy of science. In fact, these are fundamental epistemological questions in the sense of the encyclopedia definition above, and they are ones crucial to the understanding of what has counted as adequate grounds for belief in the history of scientific explanation.

There is a second reason to pause before assuming that traditional philosophy has an adequate grasp of the nature of epistemology. Sociologists of knowledge have pointed to the benefits to be gained from a kind of "externalist" understanding of epistemologies that raises skeptical questions about the adequacy of philosophers' "internalist" understandings—to borrow a contrast from the history of science. The sociologists argue that epistemologies are best understood as historically situated strategies for justifying belief and that the dominant ones in mainstream philosophy of science fail to consider important questions about the "scientific causes" of generally accepted beliefs, including those in the history of science (Bloor, 1977; Latour, 1987; Latour & Woolgar, 1979). They criticize the assumption that only false beliefs have social causes, and they call for accounts of the social conditions generating historically situated true beliefs as well as false ones. These sociologies of knowledge have all the flaws of functionalist accounts; they implicitly assume as grounds for their own account precisely the epistemology they so effectively undermine; and they are bereft of any hint of feminist consciousness.[4] Nevertheless, one can recognize the value for feminist theorists of an approach that opens the way to locating within history the origins of true belief as well as false belief and also epistemological agendas within science. Justificatory strategies have authors and intended and actual audiences. How do assumptions about the gender of audiences shape traditional epistemological agendas and claims? How should feminists reread epistemologies "against the grain"? How should such sociological and textual understandings of epistemologies shape feminist theories of knowledge?

This is perhaps the best place to point out that there have been at least three main epistemologies developed in response to problems, such as those identified earlier, arising from the feminist social science and biological research. Each draws on the resources of an androcentric tradition and attempts to transform the paternal discourse into one useful for feminist ends. What I have called "feminist empiricism" seeks to account for androcentric bias, women as knowers, and more objective but politically guided inquiry while retaining as much as possible of the traditional epistemology of science. What their authors call the "feminist standpoint epistemologies" draw on the theoretically richer resources of Marxist epistemology to explain these three anomalies in ways that avoid the problems encountered by feminist empiricism. But postmodernist critics argue that this epistemology founders on the wrecks of no longer viable enlightenment projects. Feminist forms of postmodernism attempt to resolve these problems, in the process revealing flaws in their own paternal discourse. I have argued that the flaws in these epistemologies originate in what they borrow from their nonfeminist ancestors and that, in spite of these flaws, each is effective and valuable in the justificatory domains for which it was intended (Harding, 1986).

Epistemological concerns have not only arisen from feminist research in biology and the social sciences but also generated it. So we have traced what is distinctive in feminist research back from techniques of evidence gathering, then to methodologies and theories, and now to new hypotheses about the potency of scientific method, about the scientific importance of women's experience, and about the positive role some kinds of politics can play in science.

One final comment is in order here. It is a problem that social scientists tend to think about methodological and epistemological issues primarily in terms of methods of inquiry—for example, in "methods courses" in psychology, sociology, and so forth. Atheoretical tendencies and excessively empiricist tendencies in these fields support this practice. No doubt it is this habit that tempts many social scientists to seek a unique method of inquiry as the explanation for what is unusual about feminist analyses. It is also a problem that philosophers use such terms as "scientific method" and "the method of science" when they are referring to issues of methodology and epistemology. Unfortunately, it is all too recently in the philosophy of science that leading theoreticians meant by the term some combination of deduction and induction— such as making bold conjectures that are subsequently to be subjected to severe attempts at refutation. The term is vague in yet other ways. For instance, it is entirely unclear how one could define "scientific method" so that it referred to practices common to every discipline counted as scientific. What methods do astronomy and the psychology of perception share? It is also unclear how one would define this term in such a way that highly trained but junior members of research teams in physics counted as scientists but farmers in simple societies (or mothers!) did not (Harding, 1986, chap. 2).

What is really at issue in the feminist method question? No doubt more than one concern. But I think that an important one is the project of identifying what accounts for the fruitfulness and power of so much feminist research. Let us turn to address that issue directly.

What Do Feminist Researchers Do?

Let us ask about the history of feminist inquiry the kind of question Thomas Kuhn posed about the history of science (Kuhn, 1970, chap. 1). He asked what the point would be of a philosophy of science for which the history of science failed to provide supporting evidence. We can ask what the point would be of elaborating a theory of the distinctive nature of feminist inquiry that excluded the best feminist biological and social science research from satisfying its criteria. Some of the proposals for a feminist method have this unfortunate consequence. Formulating this question directs one to attempt to identify the characteristics that distinguish the most illuminating examples of feminist research.

I shall suggest three such features. By no means do I intend for this list to be exhaustive. We are able to recognize these features only after examples of them have been produced and found fruitful. As research continues, we will surely identify additional characteristics that expand our understandings of what makes feminist research explanatorily so powerful. No doubt we will also revise our understandings of the significance of the three to which I draw attention. My point is not to provide a definitive answer to the title question of this section but to show that this historical approach is the best strategy if we wish to account for the distinctive power of feminist research. Although these features have consequences for the selection of research methods, there is no good reason to call them methods.

THE "DISCOVERY" OF GENDER AND ITS CONSEQUENCES

It is tempting to think that what is novel in feminist research is the study of women or perhaps even of females. It is certainly true that women's "natures" and habits frequently have been ignored in biological and social science research and that much recent inquiry compensates for this lack. However, as Engels, Darwin, Freud, and a vast array of other researchers have in fact studied women and females—albeit partially and imperfectly—this cannot in itself be a distinguishing feature of feminist inquiry.[5]

However, it is indeed novel to analyze gender. The idea of a systematic social construction of masculinity and femininity that is little, if at all, constrained by biology is very recent. One might even claim that contemporary feminism has "discovered" gender in the sense that we can now see it everywhere, infusing daily beliefs and behaviors that were heretofore thought to be gender neutral. In board rooms and bedrooms, urban architecture and suburban developments, virtually everywhere and any time we can observe, the powerful presence and vast consequences of gender now appear in plain sight. Moreover, feminist accounts examine gender critically. They ask how gender—and, especially, tensions between its individual, structural, and symbolic expressions— accounts for women's oppression (Harding, 1986, chap. 2). They also ask how gendered beliefs provide lenses through which researchers in biology and social science have seen the world. That is, gender appears as a variable in history, other cultures, the economy, etc. But, like class and race, it is also an analytic category within scientific and popular thought and through which biological and social patterns are understood. So, feminist research is distinctive in its focus on gender as a variable and an analytic category and in its critical stance toward gender.

Does this special subject matter of feminist inquiry have consequences for choices of methods of inquiry? Traditional philosophies of science often try to separate ontological assumptions about the appropriate domain of inquiry from issues about methods of inquiry. Yet one can note that behaviorists' insistence that the proper subject matter of psychology is human "matter in motion"—not the mental states hiding out in the "black boxes" of our minds—leads them to develop distinctive research designs elaborating their notions of experimental method. Certainly, the shifts in subject matters characteristic of feminist research have implications for method selection even if one cannot understand what is so powerful in feminist research by turning first to its methods.

WOMEN'S EXPERIENCES
AS A SCIENTIFIC RESOURCE

Reflection on this "discovery" of gender leads to the observation that gender—masculinity as well as femininity—has become a problem requiring explanation primarily from the perspective of women's experiences. A second distinctive feature of feminist research is that it generates its problematics from the perspective of women's experiences. It also uses these experiences as a significant indicator of the "reality" against which hypotheses are tested. It has designed research *for women* that is intended to provide explanations of social and biological phenomena that women want and need (Smith, 1979). The questions that men have wanted answered all too often have arisen from desires to pacify, control, exploit, or manipulate women and to glorify forms of masculinity by understanding women as different from, less than, or a deviant form of men. Frequently, mainstream social science and biology have provided welfare departments, manufacturers, advertisers, psychiatrists, the medical establishment and the judicial system with answers to questions that puzzle men in these institutions rather than to the questions women need answered to participate more fully and have their interests addressed in policy decisions. As sociologist Dorothy Smith (1979) points out, social science all too often works up everyday life into the conceptual forms necessary for administrative and managerial forms of ruling: Its questions are administrative/ managerial ones.

In contrast, feminist inquiry asks questions that originate in women's experiences. Davis (1971) asks why black women's important role in the family and the black family's in black culture are either invisible or distorted in the thinking of white (male) policymakers, black male theorists, and white feminist theorists.[6] Gilligan (1982) asks why male theorists have been unable to see women's moral reasoning as valuable. Kelly-Gadol (1976) asks if women really did share in the "human progress" taken to characterize the Renaissance. Hubbard (1983) asks if it is really true, as mainstream interpretations of evolutionary theory would lead one to believe, that only men have evolved. Women's perspectives on our own experiences provide important empirical and theoretical resources for feminist research. Within various different feminist theoretical frameworks, they generate research problems and the hypotheses and concepts that guide research. They also serve as a resource for the design of research projects, the collection and interpretation of data, and the construction of evidence.[7]

Is the selection of problematics part of scientific method? On the one hand, traditional scientists and philosophers will prohibit the inclusion of these parts of the processes of science "inside science proper," but that is only because they have insisted on a rigid distinction between contexts of discovery that are outside the domain of control by scientific method and contexts of justification where method is supposed to rule. This distinction is no longer useful for delimiting the area where we should set in motion objectivity-producing procedures, as it is clear that we need to develop strategies for eliminating the distortions in the results of inquiry that originate in the partial and often perverse problematics emerging from the context of discovery. Restriction of "science proper" to what happens in the contexts of justification supports only mystifying understandings of how science has proceeded in history. In reaction to this tendency, it is tempting to assert that these features of science are part of its method.

On the other hand, I have been arguing that there is no good reason to appropriate under the label of method every important feature of the scientific process. How hypotheses arrive at the starting gate of "science proper" to be tested empirically turns out to make a difference to the results of inquiry. Therefore, this process must be critically examined along with everything else contributing to the selection of evidence for or against the maps of the world that the sciences provide. We have identified here another distinctive feature of feminist inquiry that has consequences for the selection of ways to gather evidence but that is not itself usefully thought of as a research method.

A ROBUST GENDER-SENSITIVE REFLEXIVITY PRACTICE

A third feature contributing to the power of feminist research is the emerging practice of insisting that the researcher be placed in the same critical plane as the overt subject matter, thereby recovering for scrutiny in the results of research the entire research process. That is, the class, race, culture, and gender assumptions and beliefs and behaviors of the researcher her/himself must be placed within the frame of the picture that she/he paints. This does not mean that the first half of a research report should engage in soul searching (though a little soul searching by researchers now and then cannot be all bad!). Indeed, a more robust conception of reflexivity is required than this. To come to understand the historical construction of race, class, and culture within which one's subject matter moves requires reflection on the similar tendencies shaping the researcher's beliefs and behaviors. Understanding how racism shaped opportunities and beliefs for black women in 19th-century United States requires reflection on how racism shaped opportunities and beliefs for white social scientists and biologists in 1987. Moreover, feminist social scientists (and philosophers!) bear gender too, so a commitment to the identification of these historical lenses in our own work—not just in the work of 19th-century theorists or of men—will also help avoid the false universalizing that has characterized some feminist work. Thus the researcher appears in these analyses not as an invisible, anonymous, disembodied voice of authority but as a real, historical individual with concrete, specific desires and interests— and ones that are sometimes in tension with each other. Because these characteristics of the researcher are part of the evidence readers need to evaluate the results of research, they should be presented with those results (see Smith, 1979). We are only now beginning to be able to elaborate the rich dimensions of feminist subjectivities, but this project promises to undermine Enlightenment assumptions that distort traditional theory and much of our own thinking (Martin & Mohanty, 1986).

Like the other features that I have proposed as distinguishing marks of the best of feminist inquiry to date, this robust reflexivity is not helpfully contained within categories of method.

Conclusion

I ended an earlier section of this chapter at a point where our search for influences on the selection of research methods had led us to methodologies and substantive theories and then to epistemologies. After considering what some of the most influential feminist research has done, we are in a position to see how deeply politics and morals are implicated in the selection of epistemologies and consequently of theories, methodologies, and methods. Many of the most powerful examples of feminist research direct us to gaze critically at all gender (not just at femininity), to take women's experiences as an important new generator of scientific problematics and evidence, and to swing around the powerful lenses of scientific inquiry so that they enable us to peer at our own complex subjectivities as well as at what we observe. To follow these directions is to violate some of the fundamental moral and political principles of Western cultures. Thus meditation on the method question in feminism leads us to the recognition that feminism is fundamentally a moral and political movement for the emancipation of women. We can see now that this constitutes not a problem for the social science and biology directed by this movement but its greatest strength. Further exploration of why this is so would lead us to a more elaborate discussion of the new understandings of objectivity that feminism has produced—a topic I cannot pursue here (Harding, 1986).

It may be unsatisfying for many feminists to come to the conclusion that I have been urging: that the search for a distinctive feminist method of inquiry is not a fruitful one. As a consolation, I suggest we recognize that if there were some simple recipe we could follow and prescribe to produce powerful research and research agendas, no one would have to go through the difficult and sometimes painful—if always exciting—processes of learning how to see and create ourselves and the world in the radically new forms demanded by our feminist theories and practices.

Notes

1. Parts of this chapter appeared in an earlier form as the introduction to Harding (1987).

2. Many of the points I make are applicable to some areas of biology as well as to the social sciences. I will mention biology in these cases.

3. See Caws's (1967) discussion of the history of the idea of scientific method and of this distinction.

4. These claims would have to be argued, of course. It is not difficult to do so. Rose (1979) and Rose and Rose (1979) have made one good start on such arguments.

5. I mention this because some traditional researchers erroneously think they are teaching a feminist course or doing feminist inquiry simply by "adding" women or females to their syllabi, samples, or footnotes.

6. Davis (1971) is just one of the theorists who has led us to understand that in cultures stratified by race and class, there is no such thing as just plain gender but always only white versus black femininity, working-class versus professional-class masculinity, and so on.

7. As I have discussed elsewhere, they do not provide the final word as to the adequacy of these various parts of research processes. Nor is it only women who have

produced important contributions to feminist understandings of women's experiences (Harding, 1986, 1987).

References

Alic, M. (1986). *Hypatia's heritage: A history of women in science from antiquity to the late nineteenth century.* London: Women's Press.

Bloor, D. (1977). *Knowledge and social imagery.* London: Routledge & Kegan Paul.

Caws, P. (1967). Scientific method. In P. Edwards (Ed.), *The encyclopedia of philosophy* (Vol. 7, pp. 339-343). New York: Macmillan.

Daly, M. (1973). *Beyond God the Father: Toward a philosophy of women's liberation.* Boston: Beacon.

Davis, A. (1971). Reflections on the black woman's role in the community of slaves. *Black Scholar, 3,* 2-15.

Fee, E. (1980). Nineteenth century craniology: The study of the female skull. *Bulletin of the History of Medicine, 53.*

Gilligan, C. (1982). *In a different voice: Psychological theory and women's development.* Cambridge, MA: Harvard University Press.

Hamlyn, D. W. (1967). History of epistemology. In P. Edwards (Ed.), *The encyclopedia of philosophy* (Vol. 3, pp. 8-38). New York: Macmillan.

Harding, S. (Ed.). (1976). *Can theories be refuted? Essays on the Duhem-Quine thesis.* Dordrecht: D. Reidel.

Harding, S. (1986). *The science question in feminism.* Ithaca, NY: Cornell University Press.

Harding, S. (Ed.). (1987). *Feminism and methodology: Social science issues.* Bloomington: Indiana University Press.

Harding, S., & Hintikka, M. (Eds.). (1983). *Discovering reality: Feminist perspectives on epistemology, metaphysics, methodology and philosophy of science.* Dordrecht: D. Reidel.

Harding, S., & O'Barr, J. (Eds.). (1987). *Sex and scientific inquiry.* Chicago: University of Chicago Press.

Hartmann, H. (1981). The unhappy marriage of Marxism and feminism. In L. Sargent (Ed.), *Women and revolution* (pp. 1-41). Boston: South End Press.

Hartsock, N. (1983). The feminist standpoint: Developing the ground for a specifically feminist historical materialism. In S. Harding & M. Hintikka (Eds.), *Discovering reality: Feminist perspectives on epistemology, metaphysics, methodology and philosophy of science* (pp. 283-310). Dordrecht: D. Reidel.

Hubbard, R. (1983). Have only men evolved? In S. Harding & M. Hintikka (Eds.), *Discovering reality: Feminist perspectives on epistemology, metaphysics, methodology and philosophy of science* (pp. 45-70). Dordrecht: D. Reidel.

Kelly-Gadol, J. (1976). Did women have a renaissance? In R. Bridenthal & C. Koonz (Eds.), *Becoming visible: Women in European history* (pp. 137-164). Boston: Houghton Mifflin.

Kuhn, T. S. (1970). *The structure of scientific revolutions* (2nd ed.). Chicago: University of Chicago Press.

Latour, B. (1987). *Science in action*. Milton Keynes, England: Open University Press.

Latour, B., & Woolgar, S. (1979). *Laboratory life: The social construction of scientific facts*. Beverly Hills, CA: Sage.

MacKinnon, C. (1982). Feminism, Marxism, method and the state: An agenda for theory. *Signs: Journal of Women in Culture and Society, 7*, 515-544.

Martin, B., & Mohanty, C. T. (1986). Feminist politics: What's home got to do with it? In T. de Lauretis (Ed.), *Feminist studies/critical studies* (pp. 191-212). Bloomington: Indiana University Press.

Rose, H. (1979). Hyper-reflexivity: A new danger for the countermovements. In H. Nowotny & H. Rose (Eds.), *Countermovements in the sciences* (pp. 277-289). Dordrecht: D. Reidel.

Rose, H., & Rose, S. (1979). Radical science and its enemies. In R. Miliband & J. Saville (Eds.), *Socialist register*. Atlantic Highlands, NJ: Humanities Press.

Rossiter, M. (1982). *Women scientists in America: Struggles and strategies to 1940*. Baltimore: Johns Hopkins University Press.

Sherif, C. (1979). Bias in psychology. In J. A. Sherman & E. T. Beck (Eds.), *The prism of sex: Essays in the sociology of knowledge* (pp. 93-133). Madison: University of Wisconsin Press.

Smith, D. (1979). A sociology for women. In J. A. Sherman & E. T. Beck (Eds.), *The prism of sex: Essays in the sociology of knowledge* (pp. 135-187). Madison: University of Wisconsin Press.

Stanley, L., & Wise, S. (1983). *Breaking out: Feminist consciousness and feminist research*. Boston: Routledge & Kegan Paul.

Werkerle, G. R. (1980). Women in the urban environment. *Signs: Journal of Women in Culture and Society, 5*:3, Supplement.

Afterword

There is only one major change I would make in "The Method Question" were I writing it today. It is occasioned by Dorothy Smith's (1989) discussion of that work in a symposium on it that appeared in the *American Philosophical Association Newsletter on Feminism and Philosophy*. There Smith contrasted the epistemological preoccupations of philosophers with practicing sociologists' concerns to figure out how to get knowledge. Sociologists have to be concerned with methods of research—with how to go about getting sociological knowledge—Smith pointed out. My criticisms of feminist attempts to specify a feminist method did not take account of researchers' needs. I responded to her argument (Harding, 1989) but since have come to see differently one issue that lay between us there.

Why shouldn't feminists appropriate and transform the notion and practices of scientific method just as we have other central elements of conventional thought and practices that we want to refashion for our projects? Although she does not put the point exactly this way, I agree with Smith about this. After all, my own research has attempted to "reoccupy" epistemology and some of its associated notions, such as objectivity (Harding, 1986, 1991, 1992). Epistemology and the search for objectivity are two preoccupations of Western modernity that have been widely criticized as linked to the coercive use of power. In her comment on my paper, Naomi Scheman (1989) showed how Descartes'

125

specification of a distinctive scientific method both birthed a new, modern subject of knowledge and simultaneously attempted to secure his authority. Aren't feminist researchers and theorists, along with racial minorities in the West, postcolonials, gay and lesbian thinkers, and the members of the other new, emancipatory social movements similarly attempting to birth new, post-Enlightenment subjects of knowledge and history and to secure a certain authority for them in the face of the coercive power of conventional authorities?

I would still make all the specific arguments of "The Method Question." We should be skeptical of "methodolatry," of the attempt to separate research methods from substantive theories and from the politics and morals that permeate both, of too narrow specifications of distinctive feminist method, and so forth. However, I would see the difficult task of figuring out how to go about generating knowledge in the natural and social sciences as, in part, producing general standards for "strong method" that can generate the less biased and more comprehensive results of research ("strong objectivity") that so many feminists and other critics of conventional research practices have called for.

References

Harding, S. (1986). *The science question in feminism.* Ithaca, NY: Cornell University Press.

Harding, S. (1989). Response (to Scheman's and Smith's "Comments"). *American Philosophical Association Newsletter on Feminism and Philosophy, 88*(3), 46-49.

Harding, S. (1991). *Whose science? Whose knowledge? Thinking from women's lives.* Ithaca, NY: Cornell University Press.

Harding, S. (1992). After the neutrality ideal: Science, politics, and "strong objectivity." *Social Research, 59,* 567-587.

Scheman, N. (1989). Commentary (on Sandra Harding's "The Method Question"). *American Philosophical Association Newsletter on Feminism and Philosophy, 88*(3), 40-44.

Smith, D. (1989). Comment (on Sandra Harding's "The Method Question"). *American Philosophical Association Newsletter on Feminism and Philosophy, 88*(3), 44-46.

10

Pain

An Issue of Gender

GAYLE GIBONEY PAGE

In a word, pain is dehumanizing. The severer the pain, the more it overshadows the patient's intelligence. All she or he can think about is pain; there is no past pain-free memory, no pain-free future, only the pain-filled present. Pain destroys autonomy: The patient is afraid to make the slightest movement. All choices are focused on either relieving the present pain or preventing greater future pain, and for this one will sell one's soul. Pain is humiliating: It destroys all sense of self-esteem accompanied by feelings of helplessness in the grip of pain, dependency on drugs, and being a burden to others. In its extreme, pain destroys the soul itself and all will to live.

Lisson (1987, p. 654)

" It is an indictment of modern medicine that an apparently simple problem such as the reliable relief of postoperative pain remains largely unsolved" ("Postoperative Pain," 1978, p. 517). The concept of pain has become a focus of scientific investigation only in the past 25 years. Despite our ability to completely eradicate pain in the vast majority of cases, the human experience of pain marches on with few signs of improvement. There are numerous studies that have documented the

127

less than adequate pain management practices of the health care professionals (Beyer, DeGood, Ashley, & Russell, 1983; Donovan, Dillon, & McGuire, 1987; Marks & Sachar, 1973; Schechter, Allen, & Hanson, 1986). These studies found that hospitalized patients of all ages suffered a great deal of pain for reasons ranging from insufficient and even nonexistent physician orders for pain medication to the complete lack of pain-relieving drug administration by nursing staff.

I propose that there is a genderization of pain, and it is promoted by the pervading androcentric philosophical belief system. This belief system drives the conduct of science, and society's acceptance of that science, and the health care practices it influences. Some aspects of pain—for example, the transmission of the electrical impulses resulting from painful stimuli, phenomena that can be observed and measured—are acknowledged and valued. However, other aspects of pain, such as the pain experienced by an individual, cannot be observed directly by another and is of little if any value from the perspective of the androcentric belief system. I use valuing to connote importance and worthiness of consideration, to be of high regard. My thesis in this chapter is that pain is an issue of gender.

The discussion supporting this thesis is in two parts. The first explores contemporary feminist critique of selected scientific beliefs and practices. The purpose of this discussion is to describe the philosophical and societal context in which research in general and pain research in particular has been and largely continues to be performed. In the second part, several empirical studies regarding pain are presented in an effort to provide research-based evidence of gender bias and the need to investigate sex-related differences in pain research.

Androcentric Science, Feminist Critique

As science theorists and gender theorists have argued, both science and gender are socially constructed categories:

> Science is the name we give to a set of practices and a body of knowledge delineated by a community, not simply defined by the exigencies of logical proof and experimental verification. Similarly, masculine and feminine are categories defined by a culture, not by biological necessity. Women, men, and science are created, together, out of a complex dynamic of interwoven cognitive, emotional, and social forces. (Keller, 1985, p. 4)

> Science is politics by other means, and it also generates reliable informa-
> tion about the empirical world. Science is more than politics, of course,
> but it is that. It is a contested terrain and has been so from its origins.
> Groups with conflicting social agendas have struggled to gain control
> of the social resources that the sciences—their "information," their tech-
> nologies, and their prestige—can provide. (Harding, 1991, p. 10)

It would follow, then, that the dominant group defines what is important in science, from delineating the problem to interpreting the findings. The projects of White, Western, elite men dominate our society,
our politics, and our sciences.

The language of science uses sexual imagery to dichotomize science
as distinctively masculine (Harding, 1986, 1991; Keller, 1985):

> Objectivity vs. subjectivity, the scientist as knowing subject vs. the objects
> of his inquiry, reason vs. the emotions, mind vs. body in each case the
> former has been associated with masculinity and the latter with femi-
> ninity. In each case it has been claimed that human progress requires the
> former to achieve domination of the latter. (Harding, 1986, p. 23)

Contemporary dichotomies include "hard" and "soft" data, "separate"
and "connected" knowing, and reason and intuition:

> All these dichotomies play important roles in the intellectual structures
> of science, and all appear to be associated both historically and in
> contemporary psyches with distinctively masculine sexual and gender
> identity projects. In turn, gender and human sexuality have been shaped
> by the projects of this kind of science. (Harding, 1986, p. 125)

The power of this language is exemplified in Colameco, Becker, and
Simpson (1983), who found that physicians attributed a component of
emotionality only to the somatic complaints of women:

> The conceptions of knowledge and truth that are accepted and articu-
> lated today have been shaped throughout history by the male-dominated
> majority culture. Drawing on their own perspectives and visions, men
> have constructed the prevailing theories, written history, and set values
> that have become the guiding principles for men and women alike.
> (Belenky, Clinchy, Goldberger, & Tarule, 1986, p. 5)

The methods employed by traditional science are intended to produce results of research that are believed to be generalizable to all populations by virtue of the extensive use of control groups and random assignment to treatment groups. Basic research regarding pain typically has used male subjects, both animal and human. Although this tradition of using males may be well-intended in terms of having a relatively even hormonal environment for experiments, it cannot be assumed that such findings are generalizable to females; indeed, recent research findings would lead one to question the validity of such an assumption. Also, several recent studies indicate that it may be necessary to consider developing different methods for relieving pain that take into account the hormonal rhythms of cycling women and perhaps even new and more effective drugs for women. Another area of research that should be pursued would examine whether and how pain inhibition systems develop in very young children and beyond menopause in women.

Empirical Studies Regarding Pain

The purpose for discussing the following empirical studies regarding pain is twofold: to demonstrate that there is, indeed, an androcentric bias in the study and management of pain in humans and to provide evidence, using findings from several recent animal studies, that studying pain in only one group, such as males, with the assumption that results can be generalized to other groups is not valid and is no longer acceptable.

THE MEDICAL MANAGEMENT
OF PAIN IN HUMANS

In general, the pain literature reporting clinical studies in humans neglects to focus on, or even analyze for sex, age, or, in the case of females, hormonal rhythms (Berkley, 1993). When these comparisons are made and reported or can be deduced from the results presented, however, a recurrent theme is that there exists a large variation in the vigilance with which pain is managed among different groups of individuals, notably with respect to age and sex. The studies presented herein reflect this variation in pain management among children as compared to adults and among females as compared to males.

Surgical Pain Management

The care of infants is an extreme and brutal example of medically subsidized abuse. Whereas the administration of intraoperative pain medication is standard practice in older children and adults, until very recently the standard intraoperative anesthetic management in young infants did not include any type of pain-relieving medication, even for major surgery such as thoracotomy and patent ductus arteriosus (PDA) closure (Shearer, 1986; Yaster, 1987). Standard practice was that neonates undergoing surgical procedures received only nitrous oxide (laughing gas) and a curare drug that induced paralysis; in essence, the neonate was somewhat awake, unable to move, and experiencing every sensation of the operation. This anesthetic regimen was felt to be sufficient for infants up to 6 months of age. Eventually, the popular press joined in expressing outrage at these practices (Fischer, 1987; Ubell, 1987). In an effort to show that denying intraoperative narcotics to the very young actually posed a physical risk to these infants, a randomized controlled trial demonstrated that neonates undergoing PDA closure who received intraoperative narcotics exhibited a reduction in the hormonal aberrations that are associated with the procedure in the absence of intraoperative narcotic administration (Anand, Sippell, & Aynsley-Green, 1987). The two important findings of Anand et al. (1987) are that it is safe to give high-dose narcotic anesthesia to critically ill neonates and that the surgical stress response is largely reversed in neonates receiving such interventions. Shortly after the publication of their landmark study, a position statement by Poland, Roberts, Gutierrez-Mazorra, and Fonkalsrud (1987) was published in *Pediatrics* citing the work of Anand et al. and others and advocating the intraoperative use of pain-relieving medication in neonates. However, Poland et al. (1987) acknowledged that there still might be situations in which anesthetic agents must be reduced or even discontinued and that the criteria used for such action should be the same as is used for older patients.

With respect to the management of postoperative pain in children, several studies document an appalling lack of care. One of the earliest writings addressing postoperative pain relief in children claimed that "pediatric patients seldom need medication for the relief of pain after general surgery" (Swafford & Allan, 1968, p. 133). Indeed, in their sample of 60 children, Swafford and Allan (1968) found that only 2 "required" pain medication, meaning that only 2 actually received any pain-relieving drugs. Subsequent literature on pain in children was essentially nonexistent until the silence was broken by Joann Eland nearly 10 years later (Eland & Anderson, 1977). Eland (1974) documented the continuing trend of inadequate pain medication administration in 25 children, aged 5 to 8 years, who were hospitalized for such diagnoses as nephrectomy, hypospadias repair, fractured femur, burns, and spinal fusion. Despite orders for 21 of the children, only 12 were medicated for pain. Eland also matched the 25 children with 18 adults for diagnosis and showed that as a group the 18 adults received 671 doses of analgesia, 372 of them narcotics, whereas the 25 children received only 24 doses, a mere 10 of which were narcotic.

Two subsequent studies that matched children and adults for diagnosis or surgery group examined the differences in medication administration practices between children and adults. Both found that children received less than one half of the analgesics administered to adults (Beyer et al., 1983; Schechter et al., 1986). Further, Beyer et al. (1983) documented that 12 children undergoing heart surgery received no pain-relieving drugs whatsoever; all were infants and toddlers. These studies expose the disparate pain treatment of children compared to adults.

In adults, McQuay, Carroll, and Moore (1988) studied the effect of opiate premedication and local anesthetic blocks on the time elapsed from surgery to first administration of an analgesic in patients undergoing elective orthopedic surgery. The preoperative regimen (consisting of either preoperative opiate or none or either preoperative local anesthetic block or none) in this prospective study was decided on by the anesthetist managing the case. It was found that significantly more men compared to women received opiate premedication or opiate premedication in combination with a local anesthetic block. Given that both opiate premedication and local anesthetic blocks resulted in a longer time to first analgesic and that significantly fewer women received this treatment, it is no surprise that women had significantly shorter times to first analgesic administration compared to men. Although the key finding of this study, that preoperative administration of opiates and local anesthetic blocks enhance postoperative pain relief, is viewed as an extremely important one, these investigators also demonstrated the double standard of treatment among women and men with respect to pain management.

The postoperative prescription and administration of sedatives in place of or as an adjunct to pain medication appears to be biased toward greater use in adult females. Calderone (1990), in a retrospective chart review of 30 male and 30 female age-matched patients undergoing coronary artery bypass surgery, found that 5 of the 30 females received sedatives but none of the males were so medicated; further, these females were given fewer doses of pain medication. Twycross (1977) also reports that a significantly greater number of female than male terminal cancer patients received anxiolytics in conjunction with their pain medication. Although it is possible that the women in these two studies requested something for their anxious feelings (this information was not provided), these findings also might be explained by sex bias in physician attitudes regarding the assessment of women's medical complaints.

Colameco et al. (1983) found that physicians presented with vignettes describing a somatic complaint judged the female patients to be significantly more emotional than the males but no less authentic or ill. A troubling thought in the Calderone (1990) study that cannot be reconciled in view of the findings of Colameco et al. (1983) is that women received less pain medication compared to men and more antianxiety agents; thus they may have been viewed as more emotional (needing anxiolytics) and because of their emotions their pain discounted. Although this supposition cannot be supported in any way, these findings do show there is cause for concern with respect to the management of pain in women. Specifically, does the view that women are more emotional "color" the perceptions of health care providers such that they might be more likely to administer anxiolytics than pain-relieving medications.

Pain Unique to Women

Cases focusing on the pain unique to women offer especially interesting issues for discussion. Childbirth and premenstrual syndrome (PMS) are two such cases.

PMS, thinly veiled as late luteal-phase dysphoric disorder, was added to the revised third edition of the *Diagnostic and Statistical Manual of Mental Disorders* (*DSM-III-R*) despite research findings that challenged the validity of this category (e.g., Laessle, Tuschl, Schweiger, & Pirke, 1990). In adding this uniquely female mental disorder, the panel of the American Psychiatric Association charged with revising the *DSM* (an all-male panel, excepting the wife of the chairperson) refused to entertain seriously dissenting arguments from female scientists that were substantiated with research findings (Faludi, 1991). PMS is now an emotional disorder, complete with a *DSM* code number. (Incidently, at the same time and in the same manner, a masochistic/self-defeating personality disorder was approved as well.)

Two widely read mid-20th-century books still advance the claim that a painful labor is the fault of the mother (Dick-Read, 1944; Lamaze, 1970). Both books lead physicians and women to expect a cycle of fear, increased muscle tension, and pain, which is interruptable only by following the training regimen prescribed by the writer. However, other studies have pointed out that childbirth still is painful even if such training regimens are followed (Melzack, 1984). Those who follow Dick-Read (1944) and Lamaze (1970) tend to blame women for their failure dare they acknowledge that their childbirth experiences are indeed painful: "Not only does the prospective mother face pain, then, but the pain itself becomes a token of failure" (Melzack, 1984, p. 322). This is especially shocking because, as Melzack (1984) reports on several studies that he and his colleagues conducted, the high intensity of pain suffered by most women in labor was exceeded only by pain reports of patients recovering from the amputation of a digit. Despite the availability of medical techniques, such as epidural blocks, that effectively relieve pain without affecting the fetus, childbirth instruction continues to promote the perception of a less than natural birth (hence a failure) when the mother desires relief from the pain of labor and delivery.

LABORATORY STUDIES OF
PAIN INHIBITION SYSTEMS IN ANIMALS

The majority of laboratory studies exploring pain inhibition systems in animals use only males. The adequacy of control group representation in the method is the key factor in making the assumption that findings are generalizable. This assumption of generalizability endures even when only males are studied, despite the obvious female-male hormonal differences and their potential impact on outcomes. It is not surprising, then, that using females is often viewed as a confound. Laboratory studies regarding pain and pain inhibition pathways are no different; male animals are typically used with the same assumption of generalizability. Only recently has this assumption been challenged, and investigators are indeed finding that females and males often differ in their analgesic response both to stress and to analgesic drugs such as morphine (Baamonde, Hidalgo, & André-Trelles, 1989; Bodnar, Romero, & Kramer, 1988).

Baamonde et al. (1989), investigating whether there were sex differences in the sensitivity to morphine analgesia, found that, for each dose of morphine, male rats exhibited more analgesia than did ovulating females (relatively high levels of circulating estrogen). In an earlier study, Banerjee, Chatterjee, and Ghosh (1983) found that there were estrous-related differences in the sensitivity to morphine analgesia in female rats; animals in late diestrus (low levels of circulating estrogen) were the most sensitive. Although both studies made important contributions to our knowledge about the metabolism of systemically administered morphine in the presence of varying levels of sex hormones, neither completely studied the effects of sex and estrous on morphine sensitivity. In Baamonde et al. (1989), the only intact (non-manipulated) females used were those in estrus, and although Banerjee et al. (1983) used intact females in all estrous phases, they did not use males. In sum, although female-male comparisons of morphine sensitivity remain incomplete, there is reason to believe that sex- and estrous-related differences in the sensitivity to systemically administered morphine exist.

Findings from several recent studies support the notion that there are sex- and estrous-related differences in analgesic responses to stress. It has been found that all animals (humans as well) have endogenous opioid systems, such that in certain circumstances, as when the animal is stressed (e.g., threatened by a predator or is exerting physically), endogenous opioids are released in some areas of the brain, and the animal becomes less sensitive or even insensitive to pain. Moreover, some drugs—for example, naloxone—when injected before the stress session block or antagonize the analgesia resulting from experiencing the stressor; that is, they prevent some or all of the analgesic effect of the stressor from developing. Romero, Kepler, and Bodnar (1988) found that the analgesia resulting from intermittent cold-water swim stress was reversed by a preswim administration of naloxone in male rats but not in the females. Further, when Romero et al. (1988) used a different pain test after administering this same intermittent cold-water swim stress procedure, they found that the females exhibited significantly less stress-induced analgesia (SIA) than did the males. Ryan and Maier (1988) used a tailshock stress paradigm in female rats, in which the animal is restrained in a plexiglass tube and small shocks (1 mA) are delivered to the tail. They found that animals with relatively high levels of circulating estrogen exhibited less SIA compared to those with low estrogen levels. (Males were not used in this study.) These studies support the emerging supposition that female and male rats differ in both the type of analgesic response to some stressors (opioid versus nonopioid) and in the magnitude of that analgesia resulting from the stressor. Further, there may be differences in the magnitude of the analgesia resulting from a stressor among female rats related to their estrous phase.

Recently, it was shown that there are sex differences in the pharmacologic susceptibility to forced swim stress-induced analgesia (SSIA) in mice. Two drugs, naloxone and dizocilpine, shown to antagonize the analgesia resulting from forced swim stress in males did not antagonize this form of analgesia in females. Partial antagonism to this SSIA could be achieved in ovariectomized females (that is, in females without circulating female hormones), and this partial antagonism was abolished with estrogen replacement. Moreover, estrogen administration to intact or castrated males did not alter the observed drug susceptibility to SSIA in these animals. These findings suggest the existence of a novel, female-specific, estrogen-dependent system of SSIA (Mogil, Sternberg, Kest, Marek, & Liebeskind, 1993).

These are just a few examples that demonstrate why the assumption no longer should be made that pain mechanisms and the response to pain-relieving drugs are the same in males and females. One cannot assume that a drug shown to be efficacious in a male subject pool will have similar effects when used in females. In view of these selected findings, the traditional view of science is open to criticism for distortion, sexism, and perhaps even an accusation of promoting "bad science" if such research continues to assume that results using male-only samples are generalizable to females.

Conclusion

I would argue that a feminist approach provides a more complete description of the phenomenon of pain. Keller (1985) writes that "actual science is more faithfully described by the multiplicity of styles and approaches that constitute its practice than by its dominant rhetoric or ideology" (p. 125). Pain, from electrical impulse to the individual experience, is a wide-ranging concept, many aspects of which are not reducible to a linear relationship of cause and effect: "A healthy science is one that allows for the productive survival of diverse conceptions of mind and nature, and of correspondingly diverse strategies" (Keller, 1985, p. 178).

Sex is no longer an optional variable for responsible pain research. No longer is it acceptable to study only males and assume that using the appropriate male control groups entitles one to claim generalizability of results to females. No longer is it acceptable to test new pain-relieving drugs in males and simply assume their efficacy in females.

References

Anand, K. J. S., Sippell, W. G., & Aynsley-Green, A. (1987). Randomized trial of fentanyl anaesthesia in preterm babies undergoing surgery: Effects on the stress response. *Lancet, 1,* 243-247.

Baamonde, A. I., Hidalgo, A., & André-Trelles, F. (1989). Sex-related differences in the effects of morphine and stress on visceral pain. *Neuropharmacology, 28,* 967-970.

Banerjee, P., Chatterjee, T., & Ghosh, J. (1983). Ovarian steroids and modulation of morphine-induced analgesia and catalepsy in female rats. *European Journal of Pharmacology, 96,* 291-294.

Belenky, M. F., Clinchy, B. M., Goldberger, N. R., & Tarule, J. M. (1986). *Womens' ways of knowing.* New York: Basic Books.

Berkley, K. J. (1993, January/February). Sex and chronobiology: Opportunities for a focus on the positive. *IASP Newsletter,* pp. 2-5.

Beyer, J. E., DeGood, D. E., Ashley, L. C., & Russell, G. A. (1983). Patterns of postoperative analgesic use with adults and children following cardiac surgery. *Pain, 17,* 71-81.

Bodnar, R. J., Romero, M. T., & Kramer, E. (1988). Organismic variables and pain inhibition: Roles of gender and aging. *Brain Research Bulletin, 21,* 947-953.

Calderone, K. L. (1990). The influence of gender on the frequency of pain and sedative medication administered to postoperative patients. *Sex Roles, 23,* 713-725.

Colameco, S., Becker, L. A., & Simpson, M. (1983). Sex bias in the assessment of patient complaints. *Journal of Family Practice, 16,* 1117-1121.

Dick-Read, G. (1944). *Childbirth without fear.* New York: Harper.

Donovan, M., Dillon, P., & McGuire, L. (1987). Incidence and characteristics of pain in a sample of medical-surgical inpatients. *Pain, 30*, 69-78.

Eland, J. M. (1974). *Children's communication of pain.* Unpublished master's thesis, University of Iowa, Iowa City.

Eland, J. M., & Anderson, J. E. (1977). The experience of pain in children. In A. K. Jacox (Ed.), *Pain: A source book for nurses and other health professionals* (pp. 453-473). Boston: Little, Brown.

Faludi, S. (1991). *Backlash: The undeclared war against American women.* New York: Doubleday.

Fischer, A. (1987, October). Babies in pain. *Redbook,* pp. 125-126, 183-187.

Harding, S. (1986). *The science question in feminism.* Ithaca, NY: Cornell University Press.

Harding , S. (1991). *Whose science? Whose knowledge?* Ithaca, NY: Cornell University Press.

Keller, E. F. (1985). *Reflections on gender and science.* New Haven, CT: Yale University Press.

Laessle, R. G., Tuschl, R. J., Schweiger, U., & Pirke, K. M. (1990). Mood changes and physical complaints during the normal menstrual cycle in healthy young women. *Psychoneuroendocrinology, 15,* 131-138.

Lamaze, F. (1970). *Painless childbirth: Psychoprophylactic method.* Chicago: Regnery.

Lisson, E. L. (1987). Ethical issues related to pain control. *Nursing Clinics of North America, 22,* 649-659.

Marks, R. M., & Sachar, E. J. (1973). Undertreatment of medical inpatients with narcotic analgesics. *Annals of Internal Medicine, 78,* 173-181.

McQuay, H. J., Carroll, D., & Moore, R. A. (1988). Postoperative orthopaedic pain—The effect of opiate premedication and local anaesthetic blocks. *Pain, 33,* 291-295.

Melzack, R. (1984). The myth of painless childbirth (John J. Bonica Lecture). *Pain, 19,* 321-337.

Mogil, J. S., Sternberg, W. F., Kest, B., Marek, P., & Liebeskind, J. C. (1993). Sex differences in the antagonism of swim stress-induced analgesia: Effects of gonadectomy and estrogen replacement. *Pain, 53,* 17-25.

Poland, R. L., Roberts, R. J., Gutierrez-Mazorra, J. F., & Fonkalsrud, E. W. (1987). Neonatal anesthesia. *Pediatrics, 80,* 446.

Postoperative pain [Editorial]. (1978). *British Medical Journal, 6136,* 517-518.

Romero, M., Kepler, K., & Bodnar, R. (1988). Gender determinants of opioid mediation of swim analgesia in rats. *Pharmacology, Biochemistry and Behavior, 29,* 705-709.

Ryan, S., & Maier, S. (1988). The estrous cycle and estrogen modulate stress-induced analgesia. *Behavioral Neuroscience, 102,* 371-380.

Schechter, M. L., Allen, D. A., & Hanson, K. (1986). Status of pediatric pain control: A comparison of hospital analgesic usage in children and adults. *Pediatrics, 77,* 11-15.

Shearer, M. H. (1986). Surgery on the paralyzed, unanesthetized newborn. *Birth, 13,* 79.

Swafford, L. I., & Allan, D. (1968). Pain relief in the pediatric patient. *Medical Clinics of North America, 52,* 131-136.

Twycross, R. G. (1977). Choice of strong analgesic in terminal cancer: Diamorphine or morphine? *Pain, 3,* 93-104.

Ubell, E. (1987, April 12). Should infants have surgery without anesthesia? *Parade Magazine,* p. 17.

Yaster, M. (1987). Analgesia and anesthesia in neonates. *Journal of Pediatrics, 111,* 394-395.

Phenomenology and Science

Anna Omery

Carol Mack

In making the day-to-day decisions that constitute reality, persons can and frequently do categorize that reality according to types of thought. Some thoughts are viewed as opinions, some as beliefs, and some as knowledge. Each of these types of thought presupposes a specific relationship between reality and the thinker. For example, the relationship between the thinker and reality in the type of thinking categorized as an opinion is usually considered tentative and equivocal and may not exist independently of the specific thinker or group of thinkers possessing it. Any one individual's political opinion, for example, may or may not exist as reality for other individuals.

For most thinkers, knowledge is a very special type of thought. To "know" something or someone is to have in one's thoughts a reality that corresponds to a phenomenon that is independent of that thought or the thinker (Pietersma, 1989). As a result, one fundamental characteristic of knowledge is that the reality it typifies can be recognized by more than just one individual. In general, the more numerous the individuals who agree to or about a specific reality, the more comfortable other individuals are likely to be in accepting that reality as knowledge.

Scientific knowledge is usually viewed as a very special class of knowledge. Generally, for knowledge to be scientific there is a very high degree of agreement by individuals concerning the reality that scientific knowledge represents. This does not mean, however, that scientific knowledge results from a kind of democratic consensus of individuals, with the reality that gets the most votes becoming the knowledge of science. Controversies exist among those individuals who are interested in generating scientific knowledge as to just what scientific knowledge is or is not.

For many individuals, knowledge is only scientific when it has passed certain rigorous standards of method. Only when a reality has been quantified repeatedly under sufficiently controlled conditions to warrant that the same reality has been counted each time is the knowledge to be categorized as scientific. Not only must scientific knowledge meet the standard of method, it must also meet the standard of being "objective." That is, the object cannot be known subjectively by the knower but, rather, can only be known after meeting the conditions of empiricism.

Critics of these standards for the validation of scientific knowledge have come from several, often competing philosophical perspectives. One of these philosophical perspectives is phenomenology, which proposes that all knowledge represents a complex reality. It, knowledge, is more than just a simple relationship between the thinker and reality. Rather, knowledge is constituted by the meanings the specific reality has for the thinker. Specific phenomenological philosophers differ as to whether or not phenomenologically driven knowledge development can or should result in scientific knowledge.

The purpose of this chapter is, then, to examine phenomenological thought on knowledge, especially its thoughts on scientific knowledge, The discussion starts with a short description of phenomenology, followed by a brief overview of certain phenomenological thinkers' (Husserl, Heidegger, Schutz, and Merleau-Ponty) beliefs regarding science as well as phenomenology's relationship with science. A proposition describing the relationship of phenomenological knowledge and scientific knowledge is then presented.

The Foundation of Phenomenological Knowledge

THE NATURE OF REALITY

Phenomenology holds that reality consists of the meanings in a person's lived experience. Humans know the world only as they experience it, only as they, through their consciousness, act upon it and interact with it. Because reality is experiential rather than either mental or material, it does not make sense to speak of a division between a "subjective" mind and the "objective" world (Kohak, 1978). Although individuals frequently think of the world as being divided into objective and subjective realities, this concept is not consistent with persons' actual lived experience.

This conception of reality differs from the positivist view of "objective" reality. To the phenomenologist, there is no reality separate from the reality of the world as available for, to, and through experience. There is no reality separate from the interaction of a person as "a perceiving, meaning-giving being" (Smith, 1989, p. 14). Reality cannot be known independent of a person's experience with all its meanings. Thus, in phenomenology, one must give up the Cartesian notion of a separation of mind and matter.

It is the lived experience (*Erlebnis*) that gives meaning to the world. Those objects and events that we perceive and interact with are meaningful to us. Humans do not passively receive sense data; rather, through our consciousness we create a world that has meaning to us (Kohak, 1978). It is in lived experience, then, that knowledge is grounded.

THE STRUCTURE OF LIVED EXPERIENCE

If knowledge is grounded in lived experience and experience *is* reality, then it is important to examine the nature and structure of lived experience. This lived experience is composed of structures that are intentional, subjective, and eidetic. Indeed, it is these structures that stand in the way of aligning phenomenological analysis with conceptual analysis regarded as the explication of the meanings of words (Llewelyn, 1985).

Intentional Structures

Lived experience has intentional structure. Consciousness (which includes perception, cognition, affection, and other conscious acts) is always consciousness of something (Husserl, 1913/1962). Thus intentionality describes a directional relationship, the full delineation of which includes an intending object, intentional consciousness, and an intended object (Chapman, 1966). The intended object is not, however, given in perception but is constituted from the perceiver's intentional synthesis and takes its meaning from this process. We do not passively receive sense data, we make a world, and the world has meaning (Kohak, 1978).

Kohak (1978) states that "it is not simply the passive presence of an object in a subject's field of vision but this *act* of perceiving, in a strong sense, that constitutes the perceived as intelligible" (pp. 122-123). Precisely, then, because of a subject's presence in the world as an *intentio*, experience is not arbitrary but intelligible; it makes sense. The intentional structure of experience reflects each person's way of being in his or her world.

Husserl refers to intentional experiences as *noetic* and uses the term to mean that they constitute experience as meaningful, that they contain meaning within themselves (Spiegelberg, 1982). He distinguishes the *noesis*, that is, the intentional act, from its object, which he terms *noema*. The noema is not a mere projection of the intending object; it is a real object that is present in the experience as the object of a noesis. This noema is primary in experience and is distinct from the pure sensory data into which the experience might be analyzed (Husserl, 1913/1962).

Subjectivity

Lived experience is also subjective and perspectival (Oiler, 1982). As Merleau-Ponty (1945/1962) stated, "All my knowledge of the world, even my scientific knowledge, is gained from my own particular point of view, or from some experience of the world without which the symbols of science would be meaningless" (p. vii). As there are different perspectives on shared events, there are different realities.

That experience is always subjective implies that there is always, in experience, an experiencing subject, an ego, or, as Kohak (1978) translates, as *I*. *I* am aware of acting, *I* am an integral part of the experience;

indeed, there is not experience without an *I*. To be aware of acting in the world, individuals are also always aware of themselves as the subject of this action (Husserl, 1913/1962). I not only *have* an experience, I experience and recognize myself as the subject of my experience.

Besides our awareness of acting and of being the subject of the act, we are aware of the experience as intentional and therefore meaningful. As Kohak (1978) states, "Experience is not a random set of happenings but a subject's way of being in his world, of coping, adjusting, interacting, which constitutes the world as a meaningful context of action" (p. 178).

In further describing our awareness of experience, Husserl (1913/ 1962) makes a distinction between immanent and transcendent acts of consciousness. Immanent acts are those of which there is immediate awareness. Husserl describes these as experiences in which the perceived and the perceiver are so intimately related that they can be separated only in abstraction. The "self-containedness" of such perceptions is characteristic of immanent acts of awarenes: "This privileged position [however] holds only for oneself and for the stream of experience to which the self is related; here only is there, and must there be, anything of the nature of immanent perception" (p. 130).

Transcendent acts of awareness, on the other hand, are acts of awareness of others' experience. In these acts, the perceiver and the perceived are presented not as a unity but as distinct (Husserl, 1913/ 1962). The awareness of these experiences does not and cannot have the same property of absolute giveness as the awareness of an immanent act. In fact, once a subject reflects on an act of consciousness, that act is no longer immediate in awareness but transcendent.

Eidetic Structures

Lived experience has eidetic structures, meaning that there are essential principles within experience that are invariant. Our direct awareness includes not only the particulars of an experience but also the necessary principles they embody. It is through the recognition of these eidetic structures that one recognizes two separately occurring experiences as being the same phenomenon. For example, because one expects a chair to have a seat and four legs, one is able to recognize a chair whether it is a ladder back or a Queen Anne style. The classic example given is that of a triangle. At the same time that we perceive a particular triangle, drawn, for instance, on a sheet of paper, we perceive the necessary principles of a triangle: that it has three sides and a certain ratio of angles. This awareness of necessary principles, or eidetic structures, is an immanent awareness, not the result of reflection but directly perceived (Husserl, 1913/1962). The belief that experience contains essences and that these essences can be perceived if we only learn to see clearly enough is a basic precept of phenomenology.

PHENOMENOLOGY AND KNOWLEDGE

Knowledge is embedded in experience. Husserl's admonition to return to the "things themselves" as the foundation of knowledge reflects the need to study the objects and events as they appear rather than theories about them. Of primary importance are phenomena, the experience of things rather than the things themselves (Cohen, 1987).

To see phenomena clearly in their essences, it is necessary to suspend preconceptions and view lived experience through fresh eyes. To accomplish this, we set aside or *bracket* our beliefs about the world so that we can understand how it is constituted as experience (Kohak, 1978). Bracketing allows a phenomenon to speak for itself rather than through concepts or beliefs about it.

Bracketing, as described by Husserl (1913/1962) does not deny the independent existence of the world. The world is there; we can all agree on that. What is more important in understanding reality is understanding subjects' lived experience. In bracketing our assumption that the world can explain experience rather than the other way around, we facilitate the kind of perception of experience that leads not just to facts but to descriptions of meaning of the phenomena that are the phenomena. We also avoid the error of preselecting phenomena as real. Our sources of knowledge need to be the data of experience as they reveal themselves to the subject.

Phenomenological Thinking on Science

Science has a relationship with modern Western society that is unparalleled in its complexity. Science has been and continues to be both deified and vilified. Phenomenological thinkers stand in the same relation to science as do other members of society. For certain phenomenological thinkers, such as Edmund Husserl, phenomenology and science stand in positive, mutual reciprocal relationship with each other. Science provides the knowledge by which reality is revealed and all other types of knowledge legitimized. Phenomenology provides the foundational philosophical infrastructure and direction for science and its knowledge. For other phenomenological thinkers, science is a misstep away from the meaningful knowledge of reality in its totality. For some thinkers, such as Heidegger, this misstep is a critical one. It leads those wishing to understand reality away from complete comprehension of the very knowledge they wish to comprehend. Phenomenology then becomes the philosophy that at the very least rescues the knower from this misstep.

HUSSERL'S THOUGHTS
ON PHENOMENOLOGY AND SCIENCE

For Husserl, phenomenology and science are inexorably paired. He believed science to be a system of knowledge connected by reasons in such a manner that each step is built upon its predecessor in a necessary sequence. Such a rigorous connection requires absolute clarity in basic insights and systemic order in building further propositions upon. This rigor is achievable only through a return to the things themselves, through phenomenology (Spiegelberg, 1984), for it is in the intuiting of the phenomena, particular as well as universal, in which all genuine knowledge finds its terminal verification.

Husserl (1954/1970) held that the scientific knowledge of the so-called exact science was flawed, for these sciences had failed to be "rigorous." Science had failed to make sure of its basic concepts. It had neglected the descriptive clarification of the immediate phenomena (Spiegelberg, 1982). In the pattern of the mathematicized natural sciences Husserl saw nothing but selective theoretic idealizations. What was required was a philosophical examination of the natural sciences' foundations.

Husserl proposed that to become truly scientific the natural sciences must begin with the phenomena and problems themselves. All studies of theories, however significant, must take a second place. The meaning and great task of these sciences was to achieve as much objectivity starting from the subjective ground of the life-world. It was the transcendental ego in equal partnership with all other egos in an intersubjective community that forms the foundation for the intersubjective, otherwise known as objective, world.

Phenomenological reduction becomes, then, the integral moment in the descriptive, analytic, and reconstructive process of the intersubjective world (Natanson, 1978). It provides for a new method of suspension of belief. It serves the purpose of obtaining phenomena that are attainable in the "naive" or "natural" attitude (Husserl, 1960). This reduction prepares us for critical examination of what is undoubtedly given, before our interpreting beliefs enter in. With the reduction we are led back to the origins of phenomena; those origins are lost in the haste of our everyday thought (Cohen & Omery, 1994). The reality of the outerworld is neither confirmed nor denied; rather, it is "bracketed" in an act of phenomenological reduction. What is left after the elimination of all ontological assumptions are the given process of human consciousness and their "intended objects." The latter now are no longer understood as objects in the outer world but as "unities of science" or "Meaning" in the "inner world of the conscious individual" (Schutz, 1970).

Forgetfulness of this origin was responsible for the intensifying crisis of science. This crisis was both internal, in its own foundations, and external, in its relations to "life" and to man with his human values and aspiration. The only way to restore the proper balance between scientific and nonscientific knowledge was to realize that science was in fact nothing but a distillate, as it were, from the fuller life-world. This was the task of philosophy, of which the sciences were the specialized branches (Spiegelberg, 1982).

Humankind's responsibility for themselves and for their culture can be satisfied only by a science and philosophy giving the fullest possible account of all claims and beliefs. The ethos of this responsibility requires that persons know about themselves and about their situation as far as that is in their power. Philosophy becomes then the only chance to secure ultimate foundations for the scientific enterprise (Spiegelberg, 1982).

Phenomenological philosophy results in rigorous science as a result of its establishment of a complete and thorough-going inventory of all eidetic structures underlying the full range of knowledge and experience. These eidetic structures include the essential meanings as the foundation of all special disciplines embracing the social as well as the natural sciences. This inventory of essence is to be established in the constitutive grounding of intentiality through the process of reduction or bracketing. The intuiting of general essences must be based on the careful consideration of representative examples, which are to serve as stepping-stones for any generalizing ideation. The results are the absolute and complete details of what can be known, or knowledge (Natanson, 1978).

For Husserl, phenomenology, now defined as the study of the general essence of consciousness and of its various structures, presupposes the conception of universal essences. It is these universal essences that constitute science. The meaning of universal propositions can be satisfied only through the admission of general essences, that is, through phenomenology. Phenomenology and science, then, are absolutely and inexorably related.

HEIDEGGER'S THOUGHTS ON PHENOMENOLOGY AND SCIENCE

For Heidegger, phenomenology and science confront each as irreconcilable, incompatible, and mutually exclusive phenomenon. For whereas phenomenology is the way to knowledge that is truth, modern science is mathematical representation and will to control. Its representations are themselves an expression of that will to subjugate. Its concepts are grasping. Its categories are catechistic (Llewelyn, 1985).

Heidegger was critical of the direction Husserl had moved in development of the philosophy of phenomenology. Husserl is interested primarily in the epistemological aspect. He seeks to answer the question "How do we know about man?" The goal is description. Heidegger, however, seeks knowledge in the "ontic" angle. The question he wishes to answer is "What is Being and what are the foundations for philosophizing and phenomenologizing in the midst of it?" Here, the goal is understanding. By emphasizing description rather than understanding (*Verstehen*) as its basis, Husserlian phenomenology was at best useless, at worst falsifying (Cohen & Omery, 1994).

As a result, Heidegger dissociated himself from Husserl's eidetic and the transcendental approaches (Spiegelberg, 1982). For Husserl, man is an entity constituted by his consciousness; for Heidegger, consciousness, even in its sublimated phenomenological form, is conversely an activity of man, constituted by him. Heidegger undertakes to shift the center of gravity of phenomenology by making human "being" rather than pure consciousness its nucleus.

Basic Themes

The basic themes of Heidegger's phenomenology, Being and time, were already formulated when Heidegger came in personal contact with Husserl (Cohen & Omery, 1994). Heidegger sought out Husserl because he agreed with Husserl that a fresh start would require identifying and neutralizing the metaphysical preconceptions that falsify the very formulations of our philosophical problems.

However, Heidegger moved rapidly away from Husserlian thought. Heidegger held that even Husserl's phenomenology was still too naively dependent on tradition and anything but free from presupposition. Husserl's phenomenology had failed in its task of phenomenological destruction to liberate us from unconscious servitude to our metaphysical past (Spiegelberg, 1984).

Heidegger came to believe that metaphysics, science, and technology had increasingly taken the place of what should properly be called ontology, or the study of Being. Truthful knowledge is for him no longer a property of propositions. Instead, knowledge is openness to Being itself. Further, truth is a process, the event in which Being opens up to man. Being and truth are, then, intimately united.

In Heidegger's (1927/1962) seminal work, *Being and Time*, Being was identified as the presencing of persons. Collective "beings" (*Dasein*) exist in a temporal historical world in which persons manifest themselves or "be." Analysis of this world does not result in a description of being as an object, as in traditional science. Rather, the being in which we are already standing is illuminated. What is disclosed is our own being, what it means to be, or Being (Cohen & Omery, 1994).

Time is also fundamental for Heidegger. He held that time does not exist apart from Being, but Being is essentially temporal. The idea of timeless and especially of eternal Being is, for Heidegger, meaningless from the start. Time is introduced as the possible horizon for an understanding of Being and, probably, the key to the understanding of Being (Heidegger, 1977).

Heidegger was convinced that individuals usually live in complete oblivion to the question of Being. As a result, the phenomena that are the foci for Heideggerian phenomenology are usually not given. Rather, they are concealed (Llewelyn, 1985). Heidegger also makes a special point of emphasizing that Being, particularly in the case of human being, is fundamentally particularized.

Heidegger (1927/1962) attempts in *Being and Time* to address both the oblivion and the particularism that lead in the traditional knowledge development that is science to untruths being accepted as knowledge. The strategy of this work is embodied in an attack on the meaning of Being by way of an analysis of the being of man. Persons are privileged entities who are concerned about their being and thus have a certain understanding of Being, however defective, from the very start. Human beings are, as a result, fundamentally "ontological" (i.e., thinking about being). It is at this point that Heidegger's new hermeneutic phenomenology is ready to take over.

Hermeneutic Phenomenology

Husserl's hermeneutic phenomenology replaced the goal of description with the goal of understanding. Understanding is achieved through interpretation, which is the articulation of understanding's disclosures (Llewelyn, 1985). Interpretation aims at the meaning of the thing interpreted. It therefore presupposes that what is to be interpreted has meaning. Hermeneutics thus uses reflective methods that go beyond mere description of what is manifest and tries to uncover hidden meanings by anticipatory devices.

Heidegger maintained, however, that the anticipations of hermeneutic interpretations are not determined by chance ideas or popular conceptions but by the "things themselves." Every interpretation of ordinary items in daily life is related to a frame of relevance that embraces it, implies a preview looking toward anticipated meaning, and requires concepts patterns for it. Hermeneutic phenomenology is a method of bringing out the normally hidden purposes of such goal-determined beings as man.

Hermeneutic phenomenology reveals the limitations of the merely scientific approach. Being-in-the-world is the basic structure of human being. Consciousness and particularly knowledge are only modifications of the underlying fundamental relationship between being and being in the world. Traditional science, or more specifically theoretical scientific activity, is here interpreted as a modification of our usual circumspect concern with our environment. It is one of the fundamental mechanisms by which we conceal our Being from ourselves. What is called for if beings are to have knowledge is destruction. This destruction is characterized as a loosening up of the hardened tradition and the removal of the cover (*Verdeckungen*) for which tradition, including scientific tradition, is held responsible. It is not phenomenology that presumes the destruction but the destruction that presupposes the requirement for the hermeneutic phenomenology, interpretation and understanding, of the original experiences.

For Heidegger, science, in contrast to art, does not discover original truth but merely develops what is already known. This modern science along with the totalitarian state is to be understood as the necessary consequence of modern technology on which science is said to be based. Science is not uneven thinking but a degeneration of "thinking" because it does not really think at all.

Rather, knowledge is the result of reflective hermeneutic thinking. For Heidegger, reflection, which is the proper task of phenomenology, cannot be described in terms of a clear and teachable method. At best it can be understand as focused thinking, thinking that loses its character of a spontaneous activity and consists instead of an acceptance of and listening to the voice of Being. No method is called on to enforce the revelation of truth. Reflection as method at best can prepare the way of truth in the thinker.

Hermeneutical phenomenology and science, then, are mutually incompatible. Heidegger repudiates both science and research. Research is the mark of modern science, which is characterized by a certain preconception of its field and its method (Heidegger, 1977). Knowing is possible only through reflective thinking by beings on Being and the ways of being-in-the-world.

SCHUTZ'S THOUGHTS
ON PHENOMENOLOGY AND SCIENCE

Scholars who explore Heidegger's thoughts on phenomenology and science often move into a close relationship with traditional hermeneutical thought. Other scholars focus on the development of Husserlian phenomenology. Preeminent in this second group of scholars was Schutz. Prior to Schutz's work, phenomenology's focus was principally individualistic. Schutz proceeded from a preliminary individualistic perspective to the direct analysis of social relationships. On the more theoretical level, Schutz gave particular attention to the theory of intersubjectivity (Spiegelberg, 1984).

His thoughts on science (Schutz, 1970) made it clear that he accepted the idea of a set of general methodological principles valid for the natural as well as the social sciences. However, he argued that the logical positivists were not at all justified in their claim that only specifically natural-science procedures constitute scientific methods. Scientific thinking is purposive thinking, and this purposiveness alone would suffice to distinguish it from mere fancying as its purpose was to realize the solution of the problem at hand.

Schutz and Intersubjectivity

The problem that Schutz (1970) sought to solve was a sociological one. He saw the sociological as an exploration of the general principles according to which persons in their daily life organize their experiences, especially those experiences of the social world. The most fundamental, yet possibly most problematic (in that there had not yet been an adequate description) of these principles was intersubjectivity.

Schutz, after a painstaking analysis, decided that Husserl's phenomenology of intersubjectivity was insufficient. He held that Husserl's transcendental phenomenology of intersubjectivity was misconceived. Schutz confined himself to what he called "mundane phenomenology," as expressed in his studies of the structures of the social life-world, without invoking the transcendental reduction. In fact, Schutz appealed for a special *epoche* or "bracketing" of the natural attitude that puts in brackets the doubt that the world and its objects might be otherwise than they appear as the main technique for securing the phenomena of such a study of intersubjectivity.

Schutz suggested that the eidetic of intersubjectivity identified through such a process of bracketing would result in a description of the phenomenon as a fundamental ontological category of human existence. He saw intersubjectivity as the temporal meanings constituted in concrete social experiences and believed that intersubjectivity was the requisite for all immediate human experience in the life-world. It was to be accepted as a phenomenon that is unquestionably given with the presentation of other individuals in their physical appearance. Through the intersubjective experience, persons give meaning to the structure of the social world. This temporal constitution of social action in concrete experiences resulted in the insights necessary for the comprehensive understanding of ourselves in relationship with other persons.

This insight as well as the resulting understanding, available to us only through the intersubjective experience, allowed for sentient meaningful others. Through the intersubjective experience, persons endow the sensory configuration of others before them with psychological life. The sensory experience of a person by another then is at once endowed with consciousness, feeling, and the like, all similar in kind to one's own consciousness and feeling.

Schutz distinguished the different types of intersubjective experience as it relates to our close associates, the social environment including our more distant and indefinitely known contemporaries, the social world of our ancestors, and the world of tomorrow of our successors. He acknowledged the "multiple realities" or "worlds" in which we find ourselves embedded, from the world of our everyday life to the world of dreams. He showed concretely how the scientific interpretation of human actions has its basis in the world of common sense, the life-world of Husserl.

Schutz and Science

For Schutz (1970), any knowledge of the world, including scientific knowledge, involves mental constructs, syntheses, generalizations, formulations, and/or idealizations that further are specific to the respective level of thought organization. However, the province of science and scientific reasoning had its own characteristic style. In contrast to the realms of fantasy and free-floating imagination, "pure science" he held had at least aims at knowledge for its own sake. As a result, science operated with its own brand of rationality. He presumed that science consisted of purposive intellectual action, followed systematically established plans, and subjected itself to rigid rules of logic and procedure (Spiegelberg, 1984).

In the process of inquiry that is science, a demarcation line between all that does and does not pertain to the problem under consideration is established. On one side of the line are the topics to be investigated, explicated, or clarified. On the other side are the elements of the scientist's knowledge, which, because they are irrelevant to the problem, he or she decides to accept without question as nonsignificant "facts."

As soon as scientists have made up their mind as to what subjects to investigate, these scientists entered a preconstituted world of scientific contemplation handed down to them by the historical tradition of their science. This preconstituted world is constituted through and by the intersubjective meanings shared by the individuals who belong to that specific scientific discipline.

The constitution of a province of meaning within a special branch of science can be summarized as follows. First, any problem emerging within a scientific field has to partake of the universal style of that field. This problem has to be compatible with the preconstituted problems, and the solution of these problems must be either accepting or refuting of them. As a result, the latitude for the discretion of the scientist in stating the problem is in reality a very small one.

In actuality, the scientific observer's decision to study the world under an objective or subjective frame of reference circumscribes from the beginning the section of the world that is capable of being studied under the scheme chosen. The basic postulate of the methodology of science, therefore, must be the following:

1. Choose the scheme of reference adequate to the problem you are interested in.
2. Consider its limits and possibilities.
3. Make the terms compatible and consistent with one another.
4. Having once accepted this sanctioned intersubjective reference, stick to it.

Schutz went on to maintain that there is an essential difference in the structure of thought objects or mental constructs formed by the social sciences and those formed by the natural sciences (Spiegelberg, 1984). The world of nature, as explored by the natural scientist, does not "mean" anything to the molecules, atoms, and electrons. The observational field of the social scientist, however, namely, the social reality, has a specific meaning and relevance structure for the human beings living, acting, and thinking therein. The constructs of the social scientist can be thought of as second-degree constructs. That is, these constructs are made by the actors on the social scene. This behavior the social scientist has to observe and explain in accordance with the procedural rules of his science.

The irreducible starting point of all social sciences is in the experiences of the conscious human being who lives and acts in the world. The scientist deals with this work in the intellectually spontaneous, yet active model of intentionality: There is no phase of aspect of human consciousness that appears in and by itself; consciousness is always consciousness of something. The forms of consciousness are tied to the content of experiences. Experience is attention "directed" upon objects whether real or imagined, material or ideal, and all such objects are intended. This is the immanent process of all experience, and the object is apperceptionally constructed in the synthesis of different "perspectives" in which the object is actually seen or remembered later in a typified fashion (Schutz, 1970).

A very great part of social science can be performed and has been performed at a level that legitimately abstracts from all that happens in the individual actor to create typifications. But this focus on operating with generalizations and idealizations on a high level of abstraction is in any case nothing but a kind of intellectual shorthand. Whenever the problem under inquiry makes it necessary, the social scientist must have the possibility of shifting the level of research to that of individual human activity. Indeed, where real scientific work is done this shift will always become possible (Schutz, 1970).

Method, then, becomes second to intersubjective agreement of the scientist as to how the problem is to be understood. From this position, methodology is not the preceptor or the tutor of the scientist. It is always his or her pupil, and there is no great master in that scientific field who could not teach the methodologist how to proceed. But the really great teacher will remember always not to forget to learn from those pupils (Schutz, 1970).

Merleau-Ponty's Thoughts on Phenomenology and Science

For Merleau-Ponty, perception is the matrix for both science and philosophy. The world, perceived and experienced with all its subjective and objective features, is the common ground for both as well. To make sure of this ground is the first task of phenomenology. The phenomenological reduction, interpreted in the sense of Husserl's phenomenological philosophy, is seen as the necessary mode for reaching the level of our primary perceptual experience in which the world constitutes itself.

Merleau-Ponty (1964) held that human beings are not the absolute source of meaning. We do not give ready-made sense *to* our experience from a transcendental position outside the world as in Husserl; rather, we make sense out of our experience from within it. Meanings are not *given to* experience but *received from* it. As a result, knowledge is only accessible through phenomenological method.

Merleau-Ponty and Science

Phenomenological description, which was for Husserl an attempt to do the "things" themselves and to give a scientifically rigorous account of them, means to Merleau-Ponty primarily a protest against science, for he understood science in the sense of an objective study of the things and of their external causal relations. Therefore, scientific knowledge is always an approximate knowledge that at best can clarify a perception and the analysis of which will never be finished, for it will always depend on the perception of the scientist (Merleau-Ponty, 1964).

Merleau-Ponty's (1964) objections to science must be interpreted against a peculiarly French conception of science, according to which science coincides with an "objective" approach for which there are only "things" in their external juxtaposition and in their causal interactions and which ignores the concreteness of lived experience and of the meanings it carries with it (Spiegelberg, 1984). In particular, this objectivism of the abstract that is traditional science breaks down in the human sciences, which cannot dispense with a consideration of subjectively lived experiences and meanings.

For Merleau-Ponty, perception constitutes the ground level for all knowledge, and its study has to precede that of all subsequent strata, such as those of the cultural world and specifically that of science. His phenomenology of perception is, then, an attempt to explore the basic stratum in our experience of the world as it is given prior to all scientific interpretation. Hence the primary task is to see and to describe as concretely as possible how the world presents itself to perception without omitting its meanings and absences of meaning, its clarities and ambiguities.

Perception emerges as the act designed to trace elementary meaning as actually already present in the world prior to our interpretations. This emphasis on meaning as discovered, not bestowed by investing acts, was a new, although not an absolute innovation.

Given the diversity with which any one experience can be perceived, Merleau-Ponty rejected the extravagance of the absolutist quest for certainty, for perception is an existential act, an act in which we are not only passively involved but also committed to by ourselves in a world that is only partly given. Because perception is always partly indeterminate, it expresses our ambiguous relation to the world.

The world is nothing but the field of our experience, and we are nothing but a certain perspective of it. As a result, the internal and the external, the subjective and the objective are inseparable. Consequentially, Merleau-Ponty favored a return to the *Lebenswelt*, the world as met in lived experience in the sense of the later Husserl. It may be that traditional science has purchased a kind of precision, but this precision has cost science dearly. Science is then limited to only one kind of knowledge, that of a certain objective schematization. The remedy for this is to confront science with the integrity of experience rather than to oppose it with a philosophical knowledge that comes from god-knows-where (Merleau-Ponty, 1978). Phenomenological reduction with its bracketing of belief in the reality of the natural world becomes for Merleau-Ponty the device that permits us to discover the spontaneous surge of the life-world. It does so by loosening our habitual ties with the world.

Intentionality now has as its main function the goal to reveal the world as ready made and already there. Apparently, no special technique is involved, merely a change in the direction of our reflection, notably from the phenomenal field to our consciousness *of* it and specifically to its temporal structure. Rather, Merleau-Ponty held that an attempt to investigate and to describe phenomena of the life-world as faithfully as possible certainly has just as much a claim to be considered research as any human enterprise that explores our world. If science must exist, it should be as a set of means for perceiving, imaging, and ultimately living, oriented toward the same truth that is established in persons by their first experiences in the world in which they live.

Phenomenological and Scientific Knowledge

In the preceding review of significant phenomenological thinkers' conceptualization of knowledge and science, differences are self-evident and apparent. Husserl and Schutz saw a potential relationship between phenomenology and science. Heidegger and Merleau-Ponty held that phenomenology and science were, and indeed should be, in opposition. Many philosophers would insist that the controversies reflected in the diversity result in a stalemate that is insoluble. It may be considered pretentious, but it seems that in all of this diversity at least one brief conclusion can be drawn.

Although phenomenology is not the whole of science, science does not exist without phenomenology. With the exception of Heidegger (and the argument could be made that he needs to be deleted from this chapter for he truly reflects hermeneutic rather than phenomenological thought), all of these thinkers see phenomenology as a philosophy that is foundational to any knowledge development. Phenomenology provides a description of meanings of lived experiences that provides the basis for any further knowledge development. This description that is the goal of phenomenology may not be the whole of the knowledge of science, but science cannot exist without this descriptive foundation.

References

Chapman, H. M. (1966). Realism and phenomenology. In M. Natanson (Ed.), *Essays in phenomenology* (pp. 244-278). The Hague: Martinus Nijhoff.

Cohen, M. Z. (1987). A historical overview of the phenomenological movement. *Image, 19*(1), 31-34.

Cohen, M. Z., & Omery, A. (1994). Schools of phenomenology: Implications for research. In J. Morse (Ed.), *Critical issues in qualitative research* (pp. 136-156). Thousand Oaks, CA: Sage.

Heidegger, M. (1962). *Being and time* (J. Macquarrie & F. Robinson, Trans.). New York: Harper & Row. (Original work published 1927)

Heidegger, M. (1977). *Basic writings.* San Francisco: Harper.

Husserl, E. (1960). *Cartesian meditations* (D. Cairns, trans.). The Hague: Martinus Nijhoff.

Husserl, E. (1962). *Ideas: General introduction to pure phenomenology* (R. B. Gibson, Trans.). New York: Collier. (Original work published 1913)

Husserl, E. (1970). *The crisis of European sciences and transcendental phenomenology: An introduction to phenomenological philosophy* (D. Carr, Trans.). Evanston, IL: Northwestern University Press. (Original work published 1954)

Kohak, E. (1978). *Idea and experience: Edmund Husserl's project of phenomenology in ideas, I.* Chicago: University of Chicago Press.

Llewelyn, J. (1985). *Beyond metaphysics.* Atlantic Highlands, NJ: Humanities Press International.

Merleau-Ponty, M. (1962). *Phenomenology of perception* (C. Smith, Trans.). London: Routledge & Kegan Paul. (Original work published 1945)

Merleau-Ponty, M. (1964). *Sense and non-sense* (C. Smith, Trans.). Chicago: Northwestern University Press.

Merleau-Ponty, M. (1978). The philosopher and sociology. In T. Luckman (Ed.), *Phenomenology and sociology* (pp. 142-160). New York: Penguin.

Natanson, M. (1978). Phenomenology as a rigorous science. In T. Luckman (Ed.), *Phenomenology and sociology* (pp. 181-199). New York: Penguin.

Oiler, C. (1982). The phenomenological approach in nursing research. *Nursing Research, 31*(3), 178-181.

Pietersma, H. (1989). The problem of knowledge and phenomenology. *Philosophy and Phenomenological Research, 1*(1), 27-47.

Schutz, A. (1970). *On phenomenology and social relations.* Chicago: University of Chicago Press.

Smith, M. C. (1989). Phenomenological research in nursing: Commentary and responses. Response: Facts about phenomenology in nursing. *Nursing Science Quarterly, 2*(1), 13-16.

Spiegelberg, H. (1982). *The phenomenological movement: A historical introduction* (3rd ed.). The Hague: Martinus Nijhoff.

Suggested Readings

Polkinghorne, D. (1983). *Methodology for the human sciences: Systems of inquiry.* Albany: State University of New York Press.

Thevenaz, P. (1962). *What is phenomenology? and other essays* (J. M. Edie, Trans.). Chicago: Quadrangle Books.

The Experience of Surgery

Phenomenological Clinical Nursing Research

MARLENE ZICHI COHEN

Phenomenological methodology, which seeks to understand another's experience, is ideally suited to research on nursing care. Nurse theorists since Nightingale (1860) have discussed the importance of understanding patients' perceived needs in order to meet these needs effectively. The meanings that patients attribute to their experiences help determine many of the needs they have and how these needs can best be met.

AUTHOR'S NOTE: The research described in this chapter was funded by the National Center for Nursing Research, Grant #1RO1NR01813, to Principal Investigator Marlene Zichi Cohen. The author gratefully acknowledges the contributions of David E. Barloon, Kathleen Mathis, Mary Alice Ray, Sally Swenson (research nurses) and Christopher Smith who all assisted with the research. The author is also indebted to Dean Geraldene Felton and Dr. Toni Tripp-Reimer for their help and support with the grant proposal and this research. An early draft of the present chapter was greatly improved by Dean Felton's thoughtful critique.

Because each patient is unique, individual patients must clarify what their perspectives (and needs) are. Several nursing theorists have stressed that only patients can reveal the meanings they create and nurses cannot assume they understand patients' perspectives. (This aspect of nursing was particularily emphasized by: Orlando, 1961; Parse, 1981; Paterson & Zderad, 1976; Peplau, 1952; Travelbee, 1971; Watson, 1979.) Nurses can help most effectively when they correctly understand patients' perspectives and their needs; as action is based on meanings, common meanings between nurses and patients will provide the most effective base for helpful nurse-patient relationships.

Given the long-standing professional consensus in nursing that understanding patients' viewpoint is important, one might expect that all nurses seek to understand patients' viewpoints and that patients see this understanding reflected in the care they receive. Although professionals have long advocated eliciting patients' perspectives, patients' descriptions reveal that they do not experience that nurses either elicit or understand their views consistently. Numerous articles reveal that this discrepancy has changed very little over time (e.g., A. F., 1929; Ammon, 1972; English, 1983; F. B., 1920; Foreigner, 1912; Hallenbeck, 1980; Hanson, 1916; Haybach, 1993; "A Hospital Experience," 1936; Illari, 1990; "A Nurse Goes to the Hospital," 1933; An Old Patient, 1901; RN, 1989).

Because patients vary in their ability to express their needs, nurses who are alert to potential needs will be quicker to respond to the earliest cues. Knowledge of patterns of needs will provide an effective base for nurses' clinical decision making. One way to obtain this knowledge is through phenomenological investigation of the essential features of experience.

The phenomenological study reported here was designed to provide an understanding of the essential structure of the experience of having surgery. Because professional and patient views have been found to differ, interviews were also conducted with staff nurses to obtain their understanding of patients' experiences and their perspectives of the care they provided. To allow fuller exploration of the research method, the findings reported here focus on the patients' perspective. Comparison of patients' and nurses' descriptions have appeared elsewhere (e.g., Cohen, Hausner, & Johnson, 1994). Because this study was funded by the National Center for Nursing Research, it also illustrates features important to obtaining funding for phenomenological studies.

Phenomenological philosophy has been applied in a variety of ways to guide research (Cohen & Omery, 1994). Various schools have developed, with differences in approaches. The goal of these phenomenological approaches is to obtain fundamental knowledge of phenomena, either the eidetic structure or the interpretation of phenomena to bring out hidden meanings, or some combination of these goals.

This research was guided by the Dutch phenomenology of the "Utrecht School," which combines features of descriptive and interpretive phenomenology. This approach, based on the phenomenology of such scholars as Langeveld, Buitedijk, and Linschoten, has been translated and applied to social science research (Barritt, Beekman, Bleeker, & Mulderij, 1983, 1984, 1985).

Preparatory Work

BRACKETING

Husserl used the Greek term *epoche* for the phenomenological reduction. The Greek term was used by the ancient Sceptics for suspension of beliefs. The phenomenological reduction is a method of suspension of belief. It serves the purpose of obtaining unadulterated phenomena that are attainable in the "naive" or "natural" attitude, the everyday, unreflected attitude of naive belief (Husserl, 1960). This reduction prepares us for critical examination of what is undoubtedly given before our interpreting beliefs enter in. With the reduction we are led back to the origins of phenomena; these origins are lost in the haste of our everyday thought.

Reduction, which Husserl divided into two stages, allows phenomena to come directly into view rather than to be viewed (and distorted) through our preconceptions because we temporarily suspend the natural standpoint (or natural attitude) (Spiegelberg, 1982). Husserl used the mathematic metaphor of bracketing for the second stage of this suspension of belief; he did not discuss in detail the first stage, which has been interpreted to mean dropping references to the individual and particular.

Prior to beginning to conduct interviews, the research nurses and the principal investigator (PI) bracketed their presuppositions by describing their own experiences with surgery. Each wrote the answers to the interview questions or discussed them with another member of the team. These tape-recorded discussions were transcribed, and the team analyzed the descriptions to ensure that preconceptions were not introduced to the informants during the study.

INTERVIEWER TRAINING

This research began with a pilot study involving phenomenological interviews with 10 informants who had had surgery (Cohen, 1984/ 1985). Prior to beginning the larger project, staff nurse interviewers worked with the PI for one year to gain requisite experience. This training began with the bracketing interviews described above. The PI and research nurses then met weekly to discuss readings about phenomenological research, interviewing techniques, and data analysis. The research nurses reviewed an audio-tape-recorded interview the PI had conducted. Each then conducted one set of interviews (i.e., initial interview and a follow-up interview with a nurse and a patient the nurse identified). This provided the research nurses experience with indepth interviewing and the analysis process. It also established contact with staff members in four hospitals who provided names of persons to interview for the larger study.

The PI listened to and discussed all these interview tapes with each research nurse to maintain standards of quality and to monitor the equivalence of interviews. This process continued throughout the project. The PI and interviewer discussed strengths, weaknesses, and alternative approaches that could be used in future interviews. Questions for follow-up interviews that would clarify and add depth to descriptions were also discussed. The research nurse training resulted in interviewers whose styles were equivalent to that of the PI. This procedure is discussed by Tripp-Reimer (1985).

Early in the training, potential sources of interviewer bias were dealt with. Assumptions and leading statements in the interviews were discussed, and alternative responses were practiced. The importance of reflecting rather than suggesting views was stressed. Research nurses also practiced helping informants elaborate and clarify their perceptions. Some examples of problematic statements and questions used by interviewers in the pilot interviews follow.

One nurse described a patient's response to his new colostomy:

NURSE: He did hold the container so we could empty it, but he didn't do it himself.

INTERVIEWER: Why did you ask him to hold it? Were you trying to get him involved?

We discussed the fact that the interviewer's questions made assumptions and were leading. The nurse did not say she asked the patient to hold the container. It would be better to ask if holding the container was done on the patient's own initiative or if the nurse had asked him to do it. Then it would be appropriate to ask why the nurse asked him to do it.

A second example:

NURSE: I always meet them over there [at the outpatient clinic] for post-op visits.

INTERVIEWER: Then they feel like they have some support.

We discussed that the interviewer assumed that this was done to provide support to the patient and his wife. It would be better to ask "Why did you always meet them there?" to better understand the nurse's rationale.

Research Design and Methods

Our aim was to understand the essential structure of the experience, that is, the meaning of the experience that transcended what would be unique to having a particular type of surgery in a particular hospital. Therefore, patients of both genders who varied in age and who had several types of surgery were interviewed to understand what was common despite these differences. The only restriction was that patients were over 18 years old, spoke English, and had general anesthesia. We recorded age, gender, education, occupation, marital status, number and age of children, type of surgery, and prior surgical and/or hospital experience for patients to determine if it affected the experience. Common themes emerged despite differences among the informants.

Patients and their nurses in four settings were interviewed. The settings were a large university-affiliated teaching hospital, a veterans' hospital medical center, a moderate-size community hospital, and a small community hospital in the Midwest. Head nurses in each of the four hospitals identified staff nurses who we might ask to participate in the research. Those who agreed to participate then identified post-operative patients they had cared for who they believed they knew well enough to be able to describe their experiences.

Informed written consent to conduct interviews after hospital discharge was obtained from the nurses and the patients during their hospitalizations. Interviews were conducted in patients' homes within 24 to 48 hours after hospital discharge, unless health status presented a problem. Nurses were also interviewed privately 24 to 48 hours after the patient's discharge to ensure that care was not affected and that the nurse's memory of the patient was clear. Delaying the interviews served several purposes. It insured confidentiality and helped decrease concerns that the information provided would affect care. It also ensured that patients would be physically and emotionally recovered enough to discuss their experiences. The short time interval following discharge ensured that memory of the experience was clear and accurate.

Phenomenological research is frequently based on informants' memory. Understanding of an experience may well be changed by events that follow. Given these considerations, the benefits of delaying the interviews outweighed the problems with this delay.

To understand the essential elements in experience, sufficient numbers of informants must be selected to provide a detailed and clear description of the experience under investigation. For this project, 24 pairs of nurses and patients (48 people) were interviewed. Nurses were interviewed about only one patient. The number needed was estimated based on the number of people needed in prior phenomenological research that obtained complete descriptions of similar experiences. For example, Kennison (1983) interviewed 43 persons (25 patients and 18 nurses) in her research comparing nurses' and patients' views of cancer. Drew (1986) interviewed 35 adults to explore their experiences with caregivers.

There is a considerable body of literature addressing standards of quality in research. As Feyerabend (1978) noted, "Every school of philosophy of science gives a different account of what science is and how it works" (p. 73). Because science is many traditions, many standards of quality exist. Cohen and Knafl (1993) reviewed literature on standards of quality and the guidelines for evaluating qualitative research. The frameworks discussed in nursing are general, with none linked to a specific approach such as phenomenology.

Barritt et al. (1983) discussed trustworthiness and rhetorical skill as standards for phenomenological research. Phenomenological descriptions ought to be clear and accurate, and a clear argument should be presented.

Accuracy was enhanced in this research in several ways. To ensure that the data were clear and accurate reflections of the informants' views, the PI provided the research nurses with training related to interviewing skills and also reviewed all interviews as the project progressed. Phenomenological philosophy acknowledges the importance of context in experience. Each research nurse kept detailed notes about the context. Conducting multiple interviews with each informant and asking informants to verify our analysis helped make the analysis trustworthy.

METHOD OF INTERVIEWING

Interviews were designed to elicit the meaning of patients' lived experience. All patients were asked the same open-ended questions used in Cohen (1984/1985):

1. Please describe your experience of surgery and hospitalization. I would like to know what was meaningful and important to you and what the experience was like for you.

2. What did the nursing staff do that was important to you? Please include both what was helpful and whatever was not helpful to you.

3. Who else was helpful to you during your experience? How were they helpful?

4. How was your experience with this interview? What suggestions do you have for changes I might make?

Nurses who had cared for these patients were asked similar questions:

1. Please describe what you know about this patient's experience of surgery and hospitalization. I would like to know what you believe was meaningful and important to him/her and what the experience was like for him/her.

2. What did the nursing staff do that was important to this patient? Please include both what was helpful and whatever was not helpful to him/her.
3. Who else was helpful to this patient during his/her experience? How were they helpful?
4. How was your experience with this interview? What suggestions do you have for changes I might make?

The interviewers clarified what the informants meant if their statements were unclear and sought to help the informants verbalize, to clarify what was meant to be sure that the meaning of the experiences was clearly understood.

The interview questions were as open as possible to ensure that the person being interviewed, rather than the interviewer, determined the content discussed. When asked to describe their experiences, patients often asked "where" they should begin. We always responded, "Begin wherever the experience began for you." Patients who had trouble getting started might be asked, "What is the first thing you think of when you think about your surgery and hospitalization?"

Reflections of what the patient said were used to encourage the person to continue. For example, one patient said, "He [the nurse] was talking about putting a tube back down into me, to get more food into me." The interviewer responded, "He was trying to get more food into you?" The patient then elaborated about feeling "scared" about the tube but that he had difficulty eating because the food was "so different" from what he usually ate.

Other commonly used probes were "Please say more about that"; "What did that mean to you?"; "How did you feel about that?"; and "How was that helpful (or not helpful)?" When informants used jargon or spoke in generalities the interviewer would ask for an example and details about exactly what was said and done.

All interviews were tape recorded, transcribed, and analyzed. After each interview, the verbatim transcription of the interview was given to the informant. The interviewer returned and asked the informant to clarify these interviews. Follow-up interviews were also tape recorded, transcribed, and analyzed. These interviews began by asking informants if they had anything to add to their description now that they had reviewed the transcripts (of the original interview) and if there was anything they did not wish to have included in the analysis. One informant asked, for example, that discussion about her divorce not be included. Both the interviewer's questions and anything the informant felt needed to be clarified or added to the description was discussed. Informants were also asked if preliminary analysis (i.e., tentative theme names) appropriately described the meaning they sought to convey. These interviews continued until each informant felt that he or she had fully described the experience.

Informants have reported that seeing their words in print and "seeing" the experience changed it for them. However, the follow-up interviews did not add new material but served to allow the informants to clarify and elaborate on what they said. Therefore, our results were not altered by the return visit. Rather, the meaning of the initial discussion became more clear.

DATA ANALYSIS

Analysis was done by the PI, with each research nurse assisting with initial content analysis. The PI listened to each tape several times and verified the accuracy of the verbatim transcriptions of each interview. Transcripts were then coded. Data were examined line by line, phrases were underlined, and tentative theme names were written in the margin. Analysis of the following passage is an example of how the data were analyzed:

> The doctor told me, he showed me in his papers from when he discharged me that he had written down in his notes that he had told me to be on six feedings. I must have forgot and I didn't pay any attention and . . . I put some of the blame on myself because I either wasn't paying attention or didn't follow up with the six feedings he told me. I went back for my appointment to see the doctor after being discharged—I think I seen him three times. He asked me at times if I had complications or problems. I told him no. I said I have a little soreness across the incision, which is common, but no complications as far as stomach problems . . . I was having diarrhea problems at times because the food was passing through me so quickly. But I thought nothing of it. I didn't even think it was related to the surgery. I thought I had the flu or something.

This passage was coded within the category "information about self-care" and illustrated patients' "need to know" in the theme "need to know and the fear of knowing."

The labeled passages were grouped according to common labels and compared with other passages. This procedure was followed for each individual informant. The interviewer discussed these tentative theme names during the second interview with each informant to ensure that the meaning the informant sought to convey had been appropriately captured.

The next step was to compare passages and themes of each informant with passages and themes of all other informants. Passages were compared both across themes and with other passages in the same theme. The analysis also discussed elements within themes. For example, there were six categories within the theme "need to know and the fear of knowing": patients discussing wanting information about the institution and procedures, preparation for the future (probable outcomes), information to deal with changed reality, information about self-care, problems obtaining information, and enough about what was required of them to determine whether the change was reasonable for them.

Patient and nurse meanings and perceived needs were also compared between the nurse and the patient for whom she cared. We examined overall themes and also whether nurses or patients discussed some material that the other did not. For example, nurses focused on technology, whereas patients often seemed unaware of or unconcerned about complex monitoring and treatments. Implications from these differences are examined elsewhere.

Themes

Three common themes emerged in patient interviews. These themes were also found in a thematic analysis of articles published in nursing journals dating back to 1900.

The first theme was the *need to know and the fear of knowing*. Although all patients wanted some information, the kind and amount of information they wanted varied tremendously. Brief hospital pamphlets or staff relating their own personal experiences with surgery was enough for some patients. Others wanted to read medical texts, see their X rays, and know other details of what would happen to them. Some informants did not want to know some details because they were afraid to know.

Patients did not always know enough to ask. The clearest example of this was the informant who did not get enough information, in a way he could use it, about his diet after his surgery for a bleeding ulcer. As the passage presented earlier showed, he did not know he should learn about changing his diet or that diarrhea might be related to his surgery.

What patients need and want to know is very individual. Johnson and others who followed her line of research found that standardized tape-recorded messages improved outcomes for surgical patients. However, different types of information effected different outcomes (Johnson, Christman, & Stitt, 1985), and effects were significant for persons who had some types of surgery but were not significant for persons who had other types of surgery (Johnson, Fuller, Endress, & Rice, 1978). Although that research demonstrated that standardized information was better than no information, differences among patients may relate to different content that individuals need and the best process for providing the information. Our research suggests that nurses need to learn from patients what each wants to know. It also suggests that nurses need to know how to convey information in a way their patients can use it. Also, because patients do not always know what they need to know, staff members need to introduce some information about which patients do not ask. This supports Orlando's (1961) idea that a patient will not benefit from information unless the nurse finds out, from the patient, more about what this information means to that patient.

Patients need to know what to expect, what will happen to them while they are in the hospital, and what might happen after their discharge. The consequences of their illness and care that will affect their daily lives are important. The experience of surgery can profoundly alter patients' everyday life-world, and they need to know how to deal with these changes. Information about upsetting procedures must be provided if it will affect the patients' life-world. Upsetting information that will not change the patients' reality is not always wanted. Another informant illustrated this difference. Although he had many questions about his surgery and its effects, he did not want to know the details of how the surgeon would remove his leg. In contrast to this, other informants did want to know details of what the surgeon would do. Clearly, patients (rather than staff members) are best able to determine what information is not wanted when it will not change the patients' reality.

The second theme was the *fear of death*. Although all patients were fearful that they might die, only some talked about this directly. Others denied fearing death while talking about death in less direct ways. One informant illustrated this fear:

> I was not really worried about the operation, or maybe I was very worried and I was thinking that maybe I would fall asleep and never wake up. [She laughs.] I was confident in the doctor, but I was also worried about things being done well. You think that something might happen, something might go wrong. They might put the wrong things in your blood—something that would keep you asleep forever—you know, unconscious. I knew a young woman who had very minor surgery and they gave her the wrong gas. It left her unconscious forever. So I thought about that. [She then abruptly changed the topic.]

During the second interview, the interviewer asked if we were correct in thinking that she had some fear of death and that perhaps it was difficult to talk about (since she had laughed during the discussion of never waking up and had changed the topic rather abruptly). She replied,

> Death—maybe I did not think about it much. I once mentioned it to my husband and he said, "Shut up." Before surgery I did go to the bank. I wanted to be sure my husband could take the money out. I didn't give that much thought. The surgery was not dangerous. I had had anesthesia before. I am in good shape, I run. Also, I had a good doctor—that gave me security. [She then abruptly changed the topic again.]

Patients feared death prior to all surgery, both "minor" and "major" surgery. These informants and others who have described fearing death prior to surgery suggested that they needed, in regard to this existential fear, to have staff members listen to them rather than talk. When patients do mention fearing death, they often do so only indirectly. It is important that nurses understand what patients are saying and provide them the opportunity to express their fears.

All patients were aware of the possibility of death. As May noted in May, Angel, and Ellenburger (1958), and these informants confirmed, those who confronted this awareness of nonbeing experienced an existence with heightened vitality and immediacy. Although we always live in a dialectical relation with nonbeing, this reality is emotionally fear-ful. Patients were not always ready to openly discuss their fears but always appreciated the opportunity to have an accepting audience when they were ready for this discussion.

The third and final common theme, *importance of caring*, was the most important. The informants spent more time talking about this theme than any other. Different kinds of caring were important. The caring shown by the staff members was very important. Staff members showed they cared by providing physical care, making sure that patients did what they needed to do (e.g., walking after surgery), and by talking. Patients were bothered when staff members were rough, cold, or patronizing or when they rushed.

Caring from loved ones was also very important. Their physical presence relaxed patients and helped them feel safe and secure. However, these and other patients and families have reported having loved ones excluded from the hospital. For example, Campbell (1975), Fagin (1962), and Martinson (1970) all reported being excluded from hospital rooms at crucial times in the lives of their loved ones. A recent survey (Whitis, 1994) found that hospital policies about family visiting vary widely. Nursing judgment significantly influenced how visitation policies were implemented. Because nursing philosophy and patients agree that family involvement is important and helpful, fulfilling this ideal in practice is indicated.

Patients also discussed sometimes feeling better when they showed they cared for others. They talked about a desire to help other patients, staff members, and their loved ones. Nurses should consider ways to involve patients in being helpful to them and others when the patients' helping would not be detrimental to their health. Patients of course require rest after surgery. However, when they are physically able to help others, this experience of helping may increase their self-knowledge, self-esteem, and self-awareness.

Implications of Understanding

The themes contained in these informants' descriptions are onto-logical truths (i.e., they are based on being or existence). No care can eliminate the need for information, the fear of death, or the need for caring relationships. However, patients found that sharing their experiences with interested persons helped relieve anxiety. When fears, doubts, and feelings were shared, patients also tested their perceptions with the nurses' reactions. Putting an experience into words changes the experience; verbalizing helps focus ideas that were not formed before.

Several informants said that they never before talked with anyone about their experience of hospitalization and that talking about it did indeed help them. Simply asking patients about their views is a powerful intervention. It enables nurses to establish rapport, provide better nursing care, and meet the needs that patients perceive. The information that nurses learn may also help them articulate what changes are needed (and why they are needed) within their workplaces so that patients can receive the high-quality care that nurses want to provide them.

Phenomenological research makes explicit ideas, assumptions, and implicit presuppositions on which we already behave and experience life (Keen, 1975). Because these presuppositions are overlooked in the natural attitude in which we live every day, this research reveals what we know (but overlook) so we are less puzzled.

Field (1981) wrote that phenomenological research "should challenge the reader to respond by saying, 'Yes, it is like this,' or 'No, I don't believe it is like that.' In responding, further understanding is developed" (p. 291). The aim of this description was to stimulate practicing nurses to better understand patients' experiences. This understanding may enable them to provide care that meets the needs of the individuals to whom they give care. If nurses could begin to see the care they deliver through their patients' eyes, this view might initiate thought, dialogue, and, perhaps, needed changes in nursing practice.

This example of one funded phenomenological research project may be useful to researchers interested in using this method to investigate clinical questions that arise in nursing. Familiarity with phenomenological methods could also facilitate more effective nursing care. Although it is generally agreed that communication is essential for effective nursing care, it is most often discussed in the context of assessing patients and establishing effective interpersonal relationships. Communication is less often viewed as an intervention. Indeed, Bulechek and McCloskey (1992) dropped the section on communication and the chapter on active listening (Helms, 1985) when they revised their 1985 *Nursing Interventions* book. The skills and principles of communication advocated for use by nurses (e.g., Arnold & Boggs, 1989; Bradley & Edinberg, 1990) are fundamental to this phenomenological method. Our experience has shown that skilled practicing nurses benefited from training and practice with these communication skills. The impact of this intervention awaits future research.

References

A. F. (1929). Heartless nurses [Letter]. *American Journal of Nursing, 29*(2), 221-222.

Ammon, L. (1972). Surviving enucleation. *American Journal of Nursing, 72*(10), 1817-1821.

Arnold, E., & Boggs, K. (1989). *Interpersonal relationships: Professional communication skills for nurses.* Philadelphia: W. B. Saunders.

Barritt, L., Beekman, A. J., Bleeker, H., & Mulderij, K. (1983). *A handbook for phenomenological research in education.* Ann Arbor: University of Michigan, School of Education.

Barritt, L., Beekman, T., Bleeker, H., & Mulderij, K. (1984). Analyzing phenomenological descriptions. *Phenomenology + Pedagogy, 2*(1), 1-17.

Barritt, L., Beekman, A. J., Bleeker, H., & Mulderij, K. (1985). *Researching education practice.* Grand Fork, ND: Center for Teaching and Learning.

Bradley, J., & Edinberg, M. (1990). *Communication in the nursing context* (3rd ed.). Norwalk, CT: Appleton & Lange.

Bulechek, G., & McCloskey, J. (Eds.). (1985). *Nursing interventions: Treatments for nursing diagnoses.* Philadelphia: W. B. Saunders.

Bulechek, G., & McCloskey, J. (Eds.). (1992). *Nursing interventions: Essential nursing treatments* (2nd ed.). Philadelphia: W. B. Saunders.

Campbell, G. (1975). Letters. *American Journal of Nursing, 75*(3), 393-395.

Cohen, M. Z. (1985). Patients' experience of hospitalization for surgery: Implications for nursing care (Doctoral dissertation, University of Michigan, 1984). *Dissertation Abstracts International, 45,* 2O99B.

Cohen, M. Z., Hausner, J., & Johnson, M. (1994). Knowledge and presence: Accountability as described by nurses and surgical patients. *Journal of Professional Nursing, 10*(3), 177-185.

Cohen, M. Z., & Knafl, K. (1993). Evaluating qualitative research. In P. Munhall & C. Boyd (Eds.), *Nursing research: A qualitative perspective* (2nd ed., pp. 476-492). New York: National League for Nursing.

Cohen, M. Z., & Omery, A. (1994). Schools of phenomenology: Implications for research. In J. M. Morse (Ed.), *Critical issues in qualitative research* (pp. 136-156). Thousand Oaks, CA: Sage.

Drew, N. (1986). Exclusion and confirmation: A phenomenology of patients' experiences with caregivers. *Image, 18*(2), 39-43.

English, M. (1983). Ordeal. *Nursing 83, 13*(10), 35-43.

Fagin, C. (1962). Why not involve parents when children are hospitalized. *American Journal of Nursing, 62*(6), 78-79.

Feyerabend, P. K. (1978). *Science in a free society.* London: New Left Press.

F. B. (1920). Nurses from a patient's standpoint. *American Journal of Nursing, 21,* 157-159.

Field, P. (1981). A phenomenological look at giving an injection. *Journal of Advanced Nursing, 6,* 291-296.

Foreigner. (1912). Leaves from a patient's notebook. *American Journal of Nursing, 13*(1), 17-20.

Hallenback, C. (1980). Open letter. *RN, 43*(6), 70-72.

Hanson, E. (1916). The personal and the impersonal nurse. *American Journal of Nursing, 16*(5), 404-408.

Haybach, P. (1993). Suddenly seeing me. *American Journal of Nursing, 93*(1), 96.

Helms, J. (1985). Active listening. In G. Bulechek & J. McCloskey (Eds.), *Nursing interventions: Treatments for nursing diagnoses* (pp. 328-337). Philadelphia: W. B. Saunders.

A hospital experience. (1936). *American Journal of Nursing, 36*(12), 1223-1224.

Husserl, E. (1960). *Cartesian meditations* (D. Cairns, Trans.). The Hague: Martinus Nijhoff.

Illari, B. (1990). Support for pregnancy loss. *Nursing 90, 20*(2), 4.

Johnson, J. E., Christman, N. J., & Stitt, C. (1985). Personal control interventions: Short- and long-term effects on surgical patients. *Research in Nursing and Health, 8,* 131-145.

Johnson, J. E., Fuller, S. S., Endress, M. P., & Rice, V. H. (1978). Altering patients' responses to surgery: An extension and replication. *Research in Nursing and Health, 1*(3), 111-121.

Keen, E. (1975). *Primer in phenomenological psychology.* New York: Holt, Rinehart & Winston.

Kennison, B. (1983). Nurses and patients: The clinical reality of sickness (Doctoral dissertation, University of Michigan, 1983). *Dissertation Abstracts International, 44,* 456B.

Martinson, B. (1970). Must it be? *American Journal of Nursing, 70*(9), 1887.

May, R., Angel, E., & Ellenburger, H. (Eds.). (1958). *Contributions of existentialism psychotherapy.* (pp. 37-91). New York: Basic Books.

Nightingale, F. (1860). *Notes on nursing: What it is, and what it is not.* New York: Appleton.

A nurse goes to the hospital. (1933). *American Journal of Nursing, 33*(9), 845-849.

An old patient. (1901). Suggestions to nurses from a patient. *American Journal of Nursing, 2*(2), 112-113.

Orlando, I. J. (1961). *The dynamic nurse-patient relationship.* New York: Putnam.

Parse, R. R. (1981). *Man-living-health: A theory of nursing.* New York: John Wiley.

Paterson, J. G., & Zderad, L. T. (1976). *Humanistic nursing.* New York: John Wiley.

Peplau, H. E. (1952). *Interpersonal relations in nursing: A conceptual frame of reference for psychodynamic nursing.* New York: Putnum.

RN. (1989). Patient first and nurse second. *Nursing 89, 19*(1), 6.

Spiegelberg, H. (1982). *The phenomenological movement* (3rd ed.). The Hague: Martinus Nijhoff.

Travelbee, J. (1971). *Interpersonal aspects of nursing* (2nd ed.). Philadelphia: Davis.

Tripp-Reimer, T. (1985). Research in cultural diversity: Reliability issues in cross-cultural research. *Western Journal of Nursing Research, 7*(3), 391-392.

Watson, J. (1979). *Nursing: The philosophy and science of caring.* Boston: Little, Brown.

Whitis, B. (1994). Visiting hospitalized patients. *Journal of Advanced Nursing, 19*(1), 85-88.

13

A Hermeneutical
Human Science for Nursing

RICHARD H. STEEVES

DAVID L. KAHN

Late one Friday afternoon, when Steeves was deeply into his field-work, he sat at the side of his informant's bed thinking about what had happened to his informant the night before. Steeves was in the midst of a study entailing intensively following 6 young men as they underwent bone marrow transplantation (BMT) at a large cancer research center. He was in his third month of practically living with these men as they struggled through their BMT.

"Hans," the informant, was having a difficult time. He had received his new marrow 60 days ago, and by Sunday morning he would be dead. Both Hans's family and Steeves were beginning to understand that—so was Hans.

AUTHORS' NOTE: We wish to thank Richard Rorty for his helpful reading of the manuscript for this chapter.

Hans looked awful. He was extremely emaciated, his liver was failing, and his abdomen was large and rounded by fluid. His skin was a strange color, red from a radiation burn that would never heal and, at the same time, jaundiced. Multiple tubes ran into and out of him: a nasograstric tube, a urinary catheter, and a mass of spaghettilike tubes attached to his central venous line.

A few weeks earlier, Hans had looked even worse. After his open lung biopsy, a hole had been cut in the space between his ribs and a chest tube had been added to his tube collection. His platelet count had been so low that he bled into the conjunctiva of his eyes, and coupled with the jaundice his eyes glowed an iridescent and strangely alien color. Now his mouth was better, but at one point his mucositis had been so bad that he could not talk or swallow the bloody saliva that gathered there.

Yesterday evening, Hans's seizures, probably due to a fungal infection in his brain, began in earnest. Between seizures Hans turned to his mother and said, "Why me? Why did this happen to me? I've been good. What did I do wrong?"

Today, Friday, as Steeves sat by Hans's bedside, he wondered how those questions could be answered. Steeves wondered what else could happen to this man, and, most of all, wondered how he could make Hans's experience understandable to himself and anyone who might read his research.

The basic problems for nurse scientists are ontological, epistemological, and practical. Nurse scientists must consider what is real, that is, what kinds of research questions can be asked, how knowledge is produced, how inquiry proceeds, and what value their research holds for practicing nurses. All of these questions are embedded, if not apparent, in the preceding situation.

A hermeneutic approach to social science has answers to all these questions. Some of these answers are clear and intuitively appealing; others might seem radical. Overall, a hermeneutic, interpretive science offers a great deal to the understanding of phenomena important to nurses, especially if the phenomena have some of the qualities of the situation described above.

The notion of a hermeneutic human science is relatively new, although religious scholars have used a hermeneutic approach for a long time in an effort to understand sacred texts; indeed, it is within a religious context that the name hermeneutics is grounded. Hermes was the Greek god charged with interpreting the actions and statements of other gods to the human world (Bleicher, 1980).

The idea of hermeneutics, an exigetic technique used by religious scholars, was taken up by philosophers concerned with understanding the meaning of human experience. The philosophers most germane to this discussion of hermeneutics are Dilthey, Heidegger, Gadamer, and Ricoeur. In their respective discourses, hermeneutics moved from a technique used for understanding religious texts to a general philosophy of how humans understand experience. Social scientists then, in a search to expand the science of human experience and constrained by a methodology too narrowly defined through analogy with the natural sciences, used hermeneutic philosophy to offer an approach to understanding the way people experience the meaning of the world and their place in it.

Although hermeneutics is as new to nurse scientists as to other social scientists, a discourse is already evident in the nursing literature (Allen & Jensen, 1990; Benner, 1985; Reeder, 1988; Thompson, 1990). The goal of this chapter is to add to this ongoing discourse, not as philosophers or theoreticians but as researchers trying to make hermeneutics work in the service of human science as done by nurses.

Our approach is to address the question "What is real?" to determine what researchers can study. Subsequently, how hermeneutic thinking might affect the research process is discussed.

What Cannot and Can Be Studied

BEING AND BEINGS

When Steeves's BMT patient cried out in the night "Why me?", behind the cry for help, behind the search for justice and cause in the world, even behind the assertion of his own unique identity was the basic ontological question "Why must I cease to be?" This question or rather its reverse "Why is there something rather than nothing?" marks the limits of hermeneutic knowledge. This, indeed, marks the limits of human understanding altogether. What is Being? Why do things come into being and then cease to be? (Which is the same as asking why there is time.) One has no conception of even the form a possible answer to these questions might take.

This is the area of thinking that Heidegger (1927/1962) takes as his own in *Being and Time*. He makes a distinction between *beings*, which are the "things" of this world (both democracy and doorknobs fall into this category) and *Being*, the fact of existence, about which one can know almost nothing. Heidegger uses a number of metaphors to talk about Being. There is no other way to talk about it, and yet the metaphors do not altogether work. The problem is that if one could talk about Being, could describe it, could clothe it in words, then it would become just another *being* in the world, another thing like loneliness, the color red, or religion. Hence one could say that Being cannot be talked about directly; it has no characteristics. It lies beyond language somehow.

Yet some metaphors that Heidegger uses are helpful. He talks of Being as a "clearing" much like a clearing in the forest, a place into which things enter and become beings. Being is a rent in the infinite nothingness surrounding beings and can be defined only by the fact that it is the absence of nothingness; an idea which makes very little sense in ordinary language. Another metaphor used by Heidegger is light. This metaphor does not quite work because light consists of particles or waves with measurable characteristics, such as intensity and hue. However, if one thinks of light only as it is experienced visually rather than as it is known scientifically, the metaphor is useful. Light is never seen; one sees only the things or beings that are illuminated by light. Without light nothing can be seen. Yet light itself is not visible. Light lies behind the existence of every being, at least visually, and yet it is not a being. The presence of light is only evidenced by the things that are illuminated. Therefore, it is impossible to talk about light; one can only talk about the things that are illuminated. Light is the space in which things come into visual being, but that space is not a physical or measurable one.

Thus at the core of reality is a huge mystery. Why there is something rather than nothing and what this Being is that makes all beings possible is unknowable and unfathomable. One could refer to this Being by other names, for example, God, appropriation (used by Heidegger, 1962/1972, in his later work *On Time and Being*), or language (as Gadamer, 1976, seems to do), but it will not become a being in the world. One is left to celebrate Being in poetry or just behold it with *Danken* (thanksgiving), as Heidegger (1954/1961) advised.

This argument may seem to have wandered far from the subject of nursing research. Yet this notion of Being is foundational to all that can be said about the hermeneutic approach to social science. The word foundational is used here with some caution because the belief that some idea, some concept, or some truth lies behind all that can be known about reality is anathema to the hermeneutic approach. This approach denies that there is anything that is universal or unchanging in the constituency of reality. Thus the argument that Being is foundational is on safe ground because only something totally unknowable could serve as a foundation for hermeneutics. In fact, Being is foundational only in that it has no characteristics and cannot be described—and therefore is a mystery.

THE CONTINGENCY OF THINGS

When an informant cries out "Why me?", even though the scientist's personal urge is to consider the ontological question, no social scientist would ever consider it within the realm of research to answer such a question. The preceding discussion was aimed not at developing a response to the informant's anguished plea but toward developing a scientific approach that would allow others to understand his experience.

Clearly, no scientific approach can be based upon a solid, immutable foundation because the foundation of the real is a mysterious, bright, open space. Recognizing this lack of a foundation forces social scientists to accept the contingency of all that is studied and prohibits certain kinds of thinking that social scientists have been wont to use, such as the urge to look for the universal in any human experience. For example, it would make the experiences of BMT patients understandable if one could refer to the "instinctual," "essential," or "universal" emotion that all humans have when facing death. What a scientific breakthrough it would be if this experience could be reduced to an "essence" characterizing the human experience of facing imminent death. This reduction would be possible only if one could subtract from the experiences of these informants all that was contingent, that is, all the specifics that are a product of the particular time, place, and person. Everything that had to do with the diagnosis, the hospital unit, the treatment process, and any other local detail must be eliminated in the search for that essential, universal experience. Indeed, this is the approach of some Husserlian phenomenologists (Knaack, 1984; Morse, 1989).

The hermeneutic approach to understanding denies this possibility. Understanding does not lie in discovering foundations or essentials even if such essentials exist. Understanding lies precisely in grasping those contingencies, those local details that constitute the situation.

The Contingency of Emotion

One of the most tempting areas in which social scientists search for essentials is that of human emotions. At first glance there seems to be nothing as basic, universal, and foundational as a strong feeling. However, as Lutz (1988) has pointed out in her study of Pacific Islanders, emotions do not spring from instinct or something basic in the human makeup but are the products of specific social situations carefully taught in every culture.

Emotions appear primitive to Westerners and are defined as such in Western culture. This definition relates to the Western notion of mind-body separation. Whereas the body is primitive, natural, and instinctive, the mind is cultured, created, and refined. Emotions are embodied ideas or thoughts expressed through the body (Rosaldo, 1989); they are outside cultural control and hence are viewed by Westerners as more primitive than ideas expressed with words.

An embodied idea is nonetheless an idea, and as such, is the product of culture. The basic rules for how to feel in social situations are passed on from generation to generation (Lutz, 1988). Specific emotions are created in face-to-face interactions and are controlled by cultural norms. Ideas do not come with being born human; they are learned. Because all ideas are created in this fashion, they are not foundational. In sum, then, ideas are contingent upon and are the products of culture, the personal histories of the participants, and the specifics of a situation. Thus it is fruitless for a researcher to look for some universal, foundational, emotional core when trying to understand the suffering of the BMT patient crying out in the night.

The Contingency of the Body

However, one could protest that there is something that is foundational, something that all humans have in common and are born with—their bodies. Bodies have characteristics that can be identified and categorized. Why are these characteristics not foundational to human experiences? A researcher could describe bodily characteristics, codify them, and eventually come to understand human experiences in terms of the bodily characteristics involved. This is an appealing idea.

However, bodies do not have innate characteristics. To appreciate this assertion, it is necessary to understand that the experience of *embodiment,* the subjective experience of having or being a body, is different from understanding the body as would a physical scientist (e.g., physiologists, Western physicians). Physical scientists view the human body as they would view a tree, a star, or a fault line; their aim is to identify the characteristics of the human body and make claims about the universality of these characteristics.

Embodiment, on the other hand, is a lived experience, and people do not view their own bodies in the same way that physical scientists view "the human body." The characteristics that are assigned to a body by an embodied person are culturally determined and are learned by a person as he or she is socialized. As Turner (1985) wrote, the body is not a foundation of reality but, rather, a powerful vehicle for the expression of a specific social reality. One's social status, ambitions, oppressions, and social identity are stamped on the body through socialization. For example, the whole idea of body size and weight is a political statement that is culturally determined and changes over time even within a single culture (Rittenbaugh, 1982).

Some people talk of embodiment in an attempt to find characteristics that are in some way foundational to all experiences. For example, Levin (1985) finds more than implied bodily metaphors in modes of speech such as "the body politic," "grasping an idea," and "being visionary." These bodily functions are viewed somehow as the source and foundation for cerebral activities.

A clearer example of Levin's view of the world is his discussion regarding the rhythm of the human gait:

> The resounding rhythms of the dancing or walking step, the step made audible by its contact with the earth, lets us *hear* the passing measure of time—and not just in our feet, but in our body as a whole. . . . We are able to undergo an experience of *time* as a whole, and it is this which grants us, in turn, an experience of our own mortality, rounding out the movement of a lifetime. (p. 268)

In this fashion, Levin moves from a basic bodily characteristic, the rhythm of gait, to a metaphysical notion concerning time passage and mortality.

Levin's notion has poetic appeal and seems to be obviously true on some level, but it is only obvious in some cultures. In traditional Confucian culture, "the body is part of the immortal vehicle of descent linking ancestors to future generations of family members and for this reason it is not to be abused by the person, who is a transient occupant" (Kleinman, 1986, p. 193). This runs contrary to the Western notion of time and a body that is finite.

This is not to say that the body can be ignored. The absence of innate interculturally consistent characteristics does not mean that the body does not exist. The point here is that the body is not foundational in any traditional sense. Because the body is separate, unique, and finite in one culture and part of the continuous flow of creation in another, a study of the characteristics of the body would tell one only about such characteristics within the context of that specific culture. Nothing that could be said about the body could be used for the foundations of culture, for the foundations of meaning.

Of course, a body is foundational in the sense that embodiment is necessary for human existence, an echo of the argument that Being is the foundation of reality. Being and embodiment are the same characteristicless, unknowable mystery; however, in this sense, embodiment implies existing as a body, not having a body. When people think about their bodies, they can describe characteristics, count toes, classify the color of their eyes, and even decide if they are fast, strong, or good-looking, but when people hold their bodies up as objects for consideration, a distance is created and the body becomes another thing in the world. The body is no longer foundational to experiences but has become an experience.

Conclusion

Nothing is foundational to human experience. All of human experience and action is contingent upon the spatial, the temporal, and, most of all, the cultural context in which it occurs. Things that seem, at first blush, to be fundamental and universal, such as having a human body or experiencing basic emotions, are really culturally specific. They seem to be universal only because they are fundamental to the Western culture in which this chapter is written and most likely read.

Despair should not be the response to the argument that one can make no foundational assertions about human experience. Relieved of the task of finding these universals and of the mandate to make predictions and prescribe interventions, the hermeneutic scientist is left with the rich texture of everyday life in all its complexity as the subject of inquiry.

TEXTS AND HORIZONS

The process that social scientists use to understand a social situation is much like the process that any human being uses to understand his or her surroundings. The way human beings understand their worlds is best described in terms of the metaphorical "horizon" depicted by both Gadamer (1976) and Merleau-Ponty (1945/1962). Human beings perceive themselves to be at the center of a world stretching in all directions that is always already present for them (Heidegger, 1927/1962). It is somewhat deceptive, however, to speak in these terms. To say the horizon of the world is present for someone is to imply a dualism that is contrary to experience. One does not experience oneself in the center of a world that has been presented; rather, one experiences oneself as being in the center of a world of which one is always already an inseparable, integral part. In the moment of experiencing, the experiencer and the world experienced are part of the same fabric.

This inseparability is at the level of Being. Understanding takes place at a different level, the level of culture; and it is understanding that concerns the social scientist. Culture allows the experience of one's horizon to be understandable. Using the principles of understanding given by their culture, people are able to map their horizons and determine which things are near and which are far, which require attention and which do not, and which are evil and which are good. Because the horizon is temporal as well as spatial, culture allows one to use the past and predict the future.

It is important to recognize that since one is born into a culture, one experiences that culture as always already there, part of the world that one sees, not as a way of seeing the world. The realization that each culture is one among many ways of seeing the world and only appears to be a part of the world is a challenge for all thoughtful people.

To compound metaphors, people can be understood to use their cultural knowledge to read their experiential horizons, temporal and spatial, as they would a text (Gadamer, 1976; Ricoeur, 1981). Actually, this metaphor of reading a text is more useful in understanding the way that scientists approach their work rather than the way that members of a culture live in their world. A text is a static thing, permanent and unchanging; like the score to a Mozart string quartet, it is open to interpretation but not to revision. What each member of a culture does is more analogous to playing jazz than playing Mozart. The text of the piece may consist of a written score, but the written notes are intended to be only a starting place from which musicians improvise. Improvisation is based on memory, mood, careful listening to other musicians in the group, a feel for the audience, and other influences often too subtle to be identified.

Steeves's BMT patient read the basics of his situation; he knew that he was dying. He had picked up on the subtle messages of those around him, remembered what he was taught life was supposed to mean, and cried out his suffering. How does a social scientist sitting at his bedside come to understand him?

Social scientists doing fieldwork are not really different from other human beings in the way they understand their social world. They read their situation and improvise social actions just as anyone else. Social scientists enter their studies carrying with them their own culture, which has always been present for them but which has expanded to include the speech and other behavioral patterns of a social scientist. In this case, the patterns of a nurse scientist were present as well, which connotes a complex and rather specific worldview.

The social scientist has a greater task than merely understanding the situation; he/she must understand the situation from the point of view of the person(s) of focus. With regard to his BMT patient, Steeves knew how to understand what was happening in the informant's room from several different perspectives. As a nurse, Steeves had been with critically ill and dying patients and was knowledgeable about the BMT process; he understood the physiology and the nursing activities required. Steeves also understood the role of family member; he had been there. However, as a social scientist, his job was to understand what was happening from the point of view of his dying informant. Taking another's point of view is not a matter of sympathy, empathy, or even a great leap of the imagination; rather, it is the process of merging one's horizon with that of another.

This merging of horizons is a learned process that requires keen observation and study. The social scientist starts from knowing his or her own horizon and incorporates the meanings of the informant's horizon into his or her own. For example, Steeves sat in the hospital room of his BMT patient and knew what it meant for himself to be there. Then Steeves watched what the patient did, listened to what he said, and learned the topography of his horizon. Steeves never left his own place in the world; he never became the other, but he was able to incorporate a portion of the informant's horizon of experiences into his own. All people go through this process occasionally when the behavior of people around them is mysterious and is important enough to require some explanation. However, when social scientists go through this process of merging horizons, they are obliged to report the end results as well as the process through which understanding was reached.

SUMMARY

The preceding argument arose from the premise that the only foundation of reality is Being, which has no characteristics or qualities. Reality, then, is experiences that are contingent, historical, changing, socially made, and socially interpreted. In their everyday lives, people merely read a situation and improvise. The human scientist, however, needs something more to hold on to in this gliding world of social relationships. Given his or her role is to study human experience, the human scientist strives to objectify what people do and say, freeze it, and make it stationary. Hence the first step in hermeneutic analysis is to convert what is said and done into a permanently recorded text. The contingency, historicity, and, in many senses, arbitrariness of the text is never ignored, but the text becomes the working ground for the study of socially constructed meaning.

How Hermeneutics Guides the Research Act

In this section, the practical question of how hermeneutic thinking guides the research act is considered. The wording of this question is deliberate and deserves some elaboration. Although hermeneutics constitutes a methodology, a knowledge or understanding of how human science proceeds, it specifies no "method" in the sense of its present use in the nursing literature. Hermeneutics has no "protocol," to use

Morse's (1991) term, no set of detailed procedural steps that predefines an order of research events, a manner of analysis (as in phenomenology), or a typical form in which the findings appear (as in grounded theory). Instead, the researcher proceeds with his or her inquiry in a pragmatic way.

Guidance in this pragmatic process comes from the same metaphors that advance the researcher's understanding of what can be studied, and there is plenty of guidance to be found, even a structure of sorts. For example, the central metaphor of texts and the interpretation of texts as a way to understand human experiences provide both a place for inquiry to begin and a goal for the process. Situated experiences are interpreted by reading them as texts, and to do so, the researcher must find some way to convert the ongoing flow of human discourse into a stable readable form. Ricoeur (1981) refers to this process as the first form of distancing. Conversations and observations made in the "field" (the social setting under study) are "fixed" in transcription.

Data collection, then, is the construction of a text. In Steeves's BMT study, some conversations with informants were audiotaped and fixed as interview transcripts. During other conversations, the tape recorder was viewed as an intrusion, and Steeves turned it off or left it outside the room. These conversations were transcribed in field notes, along with other written descriptions of the setting and activities observed. (A thorough discussion of these latter descriptions would be tangential at this point; however, we do not mean to minimize them.)

As Steeves encountered the horizons of his BMT patient, he participated in the ongoing discourse, interpreted that discourse, and incorporated the resulting interpretations into his own understanding of the situation. Clearly though, Steeves was in a very different position from his patient's, one that allowed him some distance to observe or, more precisely, to reflect on the flow of discourse around him. This position or stance, that of the participant observer, added another layer to the text constructed in the field. The reflections of participant observers about their participation, meaning making, and emerging understanding of the situation are fixed in writing as they occur.

Thus the end result of fieldwork, the gathering of data, is a multi-layered, distanced, symbolic text concerning the meaning of the human experiences under inquiry. Obviously, this text is an interpretation (there is no such thing as "raw data"), and it is in a readable, although somewhat chaotic form. Indeed, a few authors have suggested that these texts should be presented exactly as they are at this point, allowing other readers the opportunity to make all further interpretations. Although this is an extreme position, Marcus and Fisher (1986) cite several interesting examples.

Our belief, consistent with mainstream (ironic as that word is if applied to hermeneutics outside the context of this discussion) interpretive science, is that to stop at this point is premature, an inappropriate abdication of the responsibility of authorship (Geertz, 1988). It is the author's responsibility to abstract the situated meanings into a more parsimonious text, one that is more accessible to a wider audience. At this point, the text includes hundreds, if not thousands, of pages of material and to ask others to begin here strains any commonsensical notion of science as a collective human activity. Others, including Ricoeur (1981), would argue that the text at this point fails to stand alone; its meaning still depends on the presence of the researcher/author.

The interpretation proceeds and another text must be constructed. The text constructed in the field—the field text—is read and reread by the researcher in attempts to understand its meaning. In this search for understanding, data analysis, the researcher may read the field text in various ways; the text is not yet a narrative that provides clear direction on how it should be read. For example, the field text can be read sequentially and then reread backwards from the present to the past; it can be organized and read in terms of "codes" or categories evident in the data or in terms of critical incidents or exemplars in the data. This process involves multiple readings in multiple ways and in no set order. During and from this process, the researcher's understanding of the experiential situation clarifies to a point at which the researcher is able to describe his or her understanding in an abstracted and parsimonious form; that is, as another interpretation in another constructed text. This text, the desired result of the whole inquiry, is meant to stand alone, addressed "to all who can read" (Ricouer, 1981). Finally, it has narrative form. In nursing research, this narrative text stands as the study findings of interest to other nurses, scholars, and practitioners.

That this process appears very straightforward is an artifact of this chapter's narrative form. The distinction between a data collection phase, characterized by the construction of a field text, and a data analysis phase, similarly characterized by the construction of a narrative text, is not so discrete. There is a natural division in the intensity of the researcher's preoccupation with and labor on the texts at the beginning and ending stages of the inquiry. In the middle, which is most of the time, the researcher works with both texts, going back and forth as they develop.

The idea of a dialectic underlies hermeneutic thinking. Like that of the text, it is a metaphor that guides the process of inquiry, and it does so on several levels. On the level at which the researcher clarifies his or her understanding of the situation as the inquiry proceeds, Kockelmans's (1975) discussion of the "hermeneutic circle" is seminal. Kockelmans (1975) argues that a dialectic approach is general to the development of all knowledge and a model for how a social scientist learns the meaning of any action or form of life. The researcher begins with a notion of what the situation under scrutiny means as a whole. With the awareness that this notion is vague, inaccurate, and tentative, more an "anticipation" of meaning, the researcher begins to examine the constituent parts of the situation. Which parts are to be examined is determined by the initial understanding of the whole. By examining the parts, the researcher's understanding of the whole is informed and adjusted. In turn, this new understanding of the whole affects the way that other parts are understood. Thus the hermeneutic circle continues.

Implied in this discussion of the hermeneutic circle is that the meaning eventually expressed by the researcher stems from the object of study itself; interpretive schemes are not imposed. "The source and criterion of the articulated meaning is and remains the phenomena" (Kockelmans, 1975, p. 84). This prohibition of interpretive schemes holds true for grand schema such as those offered by Sigmund Freud, Karl Marx, or Martha Rogers, as well as for those more limited in scope. Instead, the researcher aspires to an "articulated meaning" that captures the perspective of the informant. For example, in Geertz's (1973) classic account of the importance of cockfighting to Balinese men, he presented his findings in the language of an anthropologist, then reminded the reader that his perspective was that of a native. After offering 16 normative scientific-sounding statements that accounted for the meaning of bets placed on a cockfight, Geertz offered this 17th statement: "The Balinese peasants themselves are quite aware of all this and can and, at least to an ethnographer, do state most of it in approximately the same terms I have" (p. 440).

This does not mean that the interpretive researcher is unconcerned with theoretical issues. The key distinction here is the word "imposed."

Going back and forth between the specifics of what is studied and a larger world of theory is another level on which the hermeneutic circle exists. This level is crucial to the production of the narrative text.

To return to the metaphor of the horizon, the hermeneutic researcher seeks to fuse horizons, not replace his or her own horizon with another. The researcher's own horizon includes concerns with theory as influenced by his or her discipline. That is, the quality of the research process depends on a "continuous dialectical tacking between the most local of local detail and the most global structure in such a way as to bring them into simultaneous view" (Geertz, 1983, p. 69). Steeves approached the study of BMT patients with a long-standing theoretical interest in suffering and meaning (Kahn & Steeves, 1986; Steeves & Kahn, 1987). Thus a portion of the findings were presented in terms of what the experiences of BMT patients revealed about finding meaning in the face of suffering (Steeves, 1992): "No one is really interested in understanding something that is totally irrelevant for himself and the society in which he lives" (Kockelmans, 1975, p. 86).

Finally, the narrative text is, after all, the researcher's interpretation of some state and portion of everyday human experience. It is in final form only to the extent that the narrative presented to a wider audience causes it to be "fixed" in time in a physical form. In that form, it simply becomes another text for readers, including the researcher him- or herself, to interpret and reinterpret. The findings of a hermeneutic study, then, are judged only in the context of the intellectual discourse it joins and creates.

Hermeneutic Social Science and Nursing Practice

In Steeves's study of BMT patients, one of the informants had been in reverse isolation for several days. He was confined to just part of his small hospital room by means of a thick, ceiling-to-floor plastic curtain. People did not enter the room without first covering themselves from head to foot with sterile garments, including a mask. Most of this patient's social contacts were carried on by shouting through the plastic curtain over the noise of the fans that were designed to maintain high air pressure in the room.

His mucositis was causing severe mouth pain, nausea, and diarrhea. He was receiving a considerable amount of medication to control these symptoms.

One morning he talked about his hallucination the night before. He had awakened and believed that he was in the woods in northern Michigan on a fishing trip. He said that "half of him" knew that there was a streetlight shining in the parking lot outside his hospital window, and half of him knew that the light was the moon in the trees. As he sat on the edge of his bed looking at the light, he noticed that someone was sitting on the bed with him: "That other guy was throwing up and had the dry heaves. I felt really sorry for him." By morning he was back together again and could talk about what had happened.

Weeks later, as he was approaching death, he talked about an experience he had had on a fishing trip after he had been diagnosed with leukemia but before he had decided to have a BMT:

> I put three lines in the water. It was still and beautiful in the morning, and I got really emotional, felt really good after being there for about 15 minutes and decided just to talk with God. I got down on my knees and prayed for a long time. It felt really good, and I stayed there another two hours and never saw another person and never caught a fish.

He knew how good life could be, and, unfortunately, while going through this BMT, he was beginning to learn how bad life could be. His idea of life at its best and at its most meaningful was a narrative about fishing.

At the time, Steeves was not a fisherman, but he understood his informant to some extent because he remembered the long trout-fishing scene in Hemingway's (1926) *The Sun Also Rises*: the cathedral-like beauty of the woods and the stream, the stillness, the careful arranging of caught fish layered with fronds. Steeves had his own literary image that he could use to understand his informant's experience.

Novels by someone like Hemingway and the literature created by hermeneutic social scientists are quite different in most of their goals, but they share at least one common goal: preventing their readers from seeing the behavior of others as strange. As Rorty (1989) stated, "The ability to think of people wildly different from ourselves as included in the range of 'us'" can be the result of "detailed descriptions of particular varieties of pain and humiliation (in, e.g., novels or ethnographies)" (p. 192). In other words, the description of the sufferings and pleasures of the BMT patient and those of Hemingway's Jacob Barnes serve to prevent us, the reader, from finding these people, and others like them, alien. We cannot help but find them more like ourselves than different because, however vicariously, we have shared their experience.

But the hermeneutic social scientist aims at more than the development of familyhood among people, no matter how lofty that goal may be. The more direct goal of social scientists, especially nurse scientists, is to offer something useful to practitioners—in this case, texts that can be used to create exemplars.

Considerable evidence has been offered that nurses understand the condition and experiences of their patients by relying on exemplars (Benner, 1984; Kahn & Steeves, 1988; Steeves, Kahn, & Benoliel, 1990). These images or narratives about exemplary patients are interpretations by the nurse that can be based on well-remembered historical incidents, compilation accounts (the experiences of more than one remembered patient), or fictional accounts (narratives that have been read or heard). Exemplars are interpretive accounts constructed by a nurse that demonstrate what is most important about an illness experience for that practicing nurse. Extensive experience with a particular type of patient is usually necessary before a nurse is able to construct an exemplar. Novice nurses who have not had the experience from which to create exemplars must rely on rules, principles, and theories often learned in formal educational settings to direct their practice.

The hermeneutic social scientist, although he or she cannot create exemplary cases for practicing nurses, can provide the texts or vicariously experienced accounts a nurse reader can use to create these exemplars. For example, one of the purposes of the BMT study was to offer to practicing nurses close personal contact over an extended period of time with six men who were undergoing bone marrow transplantation. There is no guarantee that nurses reading the account of these men will be able to create with it exemplars that will change their practice when they come in contact with patients similar to these. The hermeneutic social scientist is in the position only to offer vicarious experience, not to prescribe, direct, or even advise. The power to convert scientific information into useful practice is completely in the hands of the practitioner, as it should be.

References

Agar, M. (1980). *The professional stranger: An informal introduction to ethnography.* New York: Academic Press.

Allen, M. N., & Jensen, L. (1990). Hermeneutic inquiry: Meaning and scope. *Western Journal of Nursing Research, 12*(2), 241-253.

Benner, P. (1984). *From novice to expert.* Menlo Park, CA: Addison-Wesley.

Benner, P. (1985). Quality of life: A phenomenological perspective on explanation, prediction, and understanding in nursing science. *Advances in Nursing Science, 8*(1), 1-14.

Bleicher, J. (1980). *Contemporary hermeneutics: Hermeneutics as method, philosophy and critique.* New York: Routledge & Kegan Paul.

Gadamer, H.-G. (1976). *Philosophical hermeneutics* (D. E. Linge, Trans. & Ed.). Los Angeles: University of California Press.

Geertz, C. (1983). *Local knowledge: Further essays in interpretive anthropology.* New York: Basic Books.

Geertz, C. (1973). *The interpretation of culture.* New York: Basic Books.

Geertz, C. (1988). *Works and lives: The anthropologist as author.* Stanford, CA: Stanford University Press.

Heidegger, M. (1961). *What is called thinking* (F. D. Wieck & J. G. Gray, Trans.). New York: Harper & Row. (Original work published 1954)

Heidegger, M. (1962). *Being and time* (J. Macquarrie & E. Robinson, Trans.). New York: Harper & Row. (Original work published 1927)

Heidegger, M. (1972). *On time and being* (J. Stambaugh, Trans.). New York: Harper & Row. (Original work published 1962)

Hemingway, E. (1926). *The sun also rises.* New York: Scribner.

Kahn, D. L., & Steeves, R. H. (1986). Suffering and threat to self: Concept clarification and theoretical definition. *Journal of Advanced Nursing, 11*, 623-631.

Kahn, D. L., & Steeves, R. H. (1988). Caring and practice: Construction of the nurse's world. *Scholarly Inquiry for Nursing Practice, 2*, 201-216.

Kleinman, A. (1986). *The social origins of disease and distress.* New Haven, CT: Yale University Press.

Knaack, P. (1984). Phenomenological research. *Western Journal of Nursing Research, 6*(1), 107-114.

Kockelmans, J. J. (1975). Towards an interpretive or hermeneutic social science. *Graduate Faculty Philosophy Journal: New School of Social Research, 5*, 73-96.

Levin, D. M. (1985). *The body's recollection of being: Phenomenological psychology and the deconstruction of nihilism.* Boston: Routledge & Kegan Paul.

Lutz, C. A. (1988). *Unnatural emotions: Everyday emotions on a Micronesian atoll and their challenge to Western theory.* Chicago: University of Chicago Press.

Marcus, G. E., & Fischer, M. M. (1986). *Anthropology as cultural critique: An experimental moment in the human sciences.* Chicago: University of Chicago Press.

Merleau-Ponty, M. (1962). *Phenomenology of perception* (C. Smith, Trans.). Boston: Routledge & Kegan Paul. (Original work published 1945)

Morse, J. M. (Ed.). (1991). *Qualitative nursing research: A contemporary dialogue* (rev. ed.). Newbury Park, CA: Sage.

Morse, J. M. (Ed.). (1989). *Qualitative nursing research: A contemporary dialogue*. Rockville, MD: Aspen.

Reeder, R. (1988). Hermeneutics. In B. Sarter (Ed.), *Paths to knowledge: Innovative research methods in nursing* (pp. 193-238). New York: National League for Nursing.

Ricoeur, P. (1981). *Hermeneutics and the human sciences* (J. B. Thompson, Trans. & Ed.). New York: Cambridge University Press.

Rittenbaugh, C. (1982). Obesity as a culture-bound syndrome. *Culture, Medicine, and Psychiatry, 6*(4), 347-361.

Rorty, R. (1989). *Contingency, irony, and solidarity*. New York: Cambridge University Press.

Rosaldo, R. I. (1989). *Culture and truth: The remaking of social analysis*. Boston: Beacon.

Steeves, R. H. (1992). Patients who have undergone bone marrow transplantation: Their quest for meaning. *Oncology Nursing Forum, 19*(6), 899-905.

Steeves, R. H., & Kahn, D. L. (1987). Experiences of meaning in suffering. *Image, 19*, 114-117.

Steeves, R. H., Kahn, D. L., & Benoliel, J. Q. (1990). Nurses' interpretation of the suffering of their patients. *Western Journal of Nursing Research, 12*, 715-728.

Thompson, J. L. (1990). Hermeneutic inquiry. In L. E. Moody (Ed.), *Advancing nursing science through research* (Vol. 2, pp. 223-280). Newbury Park, CA: Sage.

Turner, B. (1985). *The body and society*. Oxford: Blackwell.

14

Passages Through the Heart

A Hermeneutic of Choice

FRANCELYN REEDER

W hat is human choice in a society where violence is commonplace and vulnerability has become reactive rather than a signpost of options? The interpretation of the experience of choice depends on the standpoint and viewpoint of the person faced with the choice.

This chapter is developed as a hermeneutic of choice and on the origins of ethical awareness. Experiential cues serve as indicators for choice in which right relationships can be discerned illuminating various right human actions that could be taken. In the existential literature, Green's (1988) viewpoint on freedom assumes there are available options to be pursued without internal or external constraint for choice to exist. This chapter focuses on the potential extreme expressions of human touch, from tender intimacy to torture, and explores what diverse paths look like in the lives of individuals who listen to and those who do not respect their human vulnerability as a source of knowledge and wisdom for choice of action. A hermeneutic of choice illuminates the role that embodiment and disembodiment play in human discernment of right action. A convincing argument is made for the private and public realms of our lives coming together by essentially *re-membering* our bodies/our selves in relation to other persons. This vulnerable relationship is the engaging journey necessary for aspiring nurses to learn the art of compassionate human acting in the world with others in response to the profession's social mandate to provide health for people (Rogers, 1970). Ultimately, a revisitation by education to the imagination as the enigmatic human faculty of embodied knowing and choosing illuminates its critical role in the creation of options (possibilities) in situations where individuals have any number and kind of actual constraints placed on their personal freedom. The imagination as a way of knowing and acting when elevated to parity with the will and intellect can provide an aesthetic option within a pedagogy for life learning ethical awareness and moral development for optimum human conduct.

The Lens: Passages Through the Heart

Similar to the process of learning to live the good life with a wise person like Socrates or Florence Nightingale, learning to live a caring life involves a long, engaging journey.

The heart is used to symbolize the whole self, the "Cor" and "ground" of one's being, manifest through reason, affection, feeling, and will. The "passage to the heart," signified by the character [関 心] is the Chinese symbol for caring. Passage to the heart for this ancient tradition involves a passage for the one caring through their own heart as they remember, anticipate, and engage bodily in caring for and with another in those moments. Living from the heart then is authenticity; it is also intentional relationship, a choice to be made.

Experientially, as anyone who has learned to care for and with another has testified, taking shortcuts on the journey to avoid the vulnerable zones with the other is not the way of committed compassionate caring. To the contrary, life struggles more often than not invite us to engage in and live in the diverse complexities and hardships facing us or our friends. An experience of being transformed through these precious though awesome passages of the heart is also voiced by many on their return. They warn that whoever desires to embark on such a journey will not find the experience a "quick study" nor one of immediate satisfaction or constant comforts or pleasures. However, a willingness and interest to learn to care in spite of these warnings are signs that one is ready and able to *begin* this journey.

To begin the journey, I am captured by the following metaphor: The place is one of yearning to gather together the wheat that has been scattered, to re-member the journey with those who have lost what was precious to them or who have lost their way through injury or blindness, confusion, or exhaustion. The journey is accompanied by those who have been wounded but still who have not fallen asleep nor given in to despair but who muster the will to engage the moment with value and flexibility, who have a certain anticipation of possibilities so needing to be fostered. These are the teachers learning too as they go on the journey through the heart to others. They are alert and awake to surprise and struggle alike, light and shadows, and most of all to the vulnerability they and others embody to wound or be wounded on the way of life. To witness someone else's vulnerability as well as your own is a sign you are *on* the journey through the heart.

A Hermeneutic of Choice

Hermeneutics is the interpretation of interpretations, expression of expressions, and making what is foreign familiar. A hermeneutic of choice is an interpretation of my own self-study and standpoint with reference to experiential cues using the body as text as I envision individuals seeing themselves situated in the world with others. From a phenomenological standpoint, the body as inhabited, experienced as being mine, serves as the definition of "embodiment." The assumption is that embodiment is experienced as the self aware of being in relationship to one's body. That being aware of one's embodiment makes it possible to recognize another person as another you. Openness and sensitivity to one's own embodiment is described as a characteristic that makes it possible to treat another as one would want to be treated in Kantean terms.

Vulnerability is illustrated as being an embodied experience crucial to passages through the heart in this hermeneutic of choice. Vulnerability as embodied presense is recognized as vital for right action in the lives of persons on the journey of becoming a professional, wise, compassionate nurse.

Vulnerability as the Ground of Choice

The *Oxford English Dictionary* (p. 329) presents a surprising definition of vulnerable. The first is

> Having the power to wound; wounding as to "throw the vulnerable darte."

The second definition is in accordance with the more usual sense of "able":

> Taken passively, that may be wounded; susceptible of receiving wounds or physical injury. Figuratively vulnerable is b. open attack or injury of a nonphysical nature; especially offering an opening to the attacks of criticism and calumny, etc. Similarly it applies to part, point, and portion as used by the poet, O. W. Holmes "There is a human subspecies. . . to a certain extent penetrative . . . It has an instinct which guides it to the vulnerable parts of the victim on which it fastens."

And last, vulnerability is expressed in *Marcella* by Mrs. H. Ward (1894) as "the inner vulnerableness, the inner need of her affection and of peace with her."

Sally Gadow (1988) takes the position that "care is the alleviation of vulnerability . . . a covenant to do so" (p. 7). She talks about discerning morally right responses and emphasizes that "only in the context of care can the overpowering of one person by another entailed in curing . . . be redeemed" (p. 7). Further, Gadow asserts that "the only means of alleviating vulnerability . . . is for us to cross the chasm . . . between the patient's intensified embodiment and the professional's disembodiment" (p. 8). In this context, obstacles to caring (alleviating vulnerability) by professionals is starkly attributed to their tendency to "learn how to disassociate themselves from one's own body in order not to empathetically recognize the patient's pain" (p. 10).

It is my position that the professional soon forgets that they also disassociate themselves in this process from the very source within of all sensibilities, affections, emotions, and will. By doing so, they unequivocally cut themselves off from the origin of right relationship to themselves, the other, and the world. The opposite path available is the discernment path of right action recognized in the present moment; it is an experience whereby a discourse of desires is awakened like a dynamic birthing process illuminating many choices toward right action. The choice involves both self and other; willingness to stay for the long haul becomes the passage through the heart offering sustaining power to be with the other as long as it takes. Professionals can thus remain embodied and alert to present desires and needs discerning the forewarning signs and avoiding becoming disembodied in situations of caring.

Historical Influences of Disembodiment

Where does this tendency to disassociate from our own body come from? Roots can abe identified in the Western philosophical emphasis on decontextualized objectivity and educational practices derived from goals to control bias (the self). The prevailing value for cognitive, discursive sources of knowledge I call here Reasons of the Head. The opposite source of knowing, which includes a broader way of learning and being in the world that has been commonly devalued, I call Reasons of the Heart, akin to embodiment. Both of these traditions have strong influences upheld by institutions and practices in the 20th century. Notably, the traditional Western view of objectivity informs the scientific disciplines and professions as they have aspired to qualify as a science. Much has been written about the cognitive, discursive pedagogical theories of teaching and learning and is not addressed here. Attention is given to the other, variously referred to as Philosophies of the Heart, Reasons of the Heart, and embodied presence. Making sense of current cries from the world can better be heard and recognized through the viewpoint of Philosophies of the Heart and promises to evoke right action from greater clarity of the human condition.

Two Possible Extremes of
Touching: A Hermeneutic of Choice

"There are different eras in the moral history of groups of people and each generation of people has to confront the basic question as to what the specific ethical imperative of the present epoch may be" (Scheler, 1974, p. 255). The signs of the times of our generation cry out for a repatterning of our most intimate relationships, where human touch ranges from the intimacy of caring (alleviating vulnerability) to the least mindful intimacy where touching turns into violence, torture, and terror (Santiago, 1990). Increasing reports by Amnesty International (1992) of torture provide evidence of the extremes to which the human person can and has been stretched, degraded, and broken. The torturer and the tortured bear minimal resemblance in their actions and purposes, but they are both of the same human species. How is this distortion possible? There are no simple answers.

The rise of violence and suicide in our society is a bizarre manifestation of the most basic need to be acknowledged, to belong, and to be known in the best sense of the word. This kind of knowing, usually thought to be the most gentle, mindful, and sensitive of touching between humans can and has changed into an explosive intense wounding of persons, a staggering disembodied action exaggerating the vulnerability of persons.

As humans, our vulnerability includes the ability to touch each other at the very heart of our selves, where self-esteem and self-worth reside. One extreme is the gentle, sensitive touching and cherishing of the whole person. This touching is considered most inclusive of the personal life and therefore to be the most ethical and the most intimate of relationships. The intimacy of knowing the other as a person with a history, unique identity with future hopes is a knowing that derives from the gentle realm of being, the realm of Reasons of the Heart. The embodied self can be recognized in the sensing, thinking, willing, reflecting actions and expressions of a person's being. Moments of "having it together" are moments of special integrity; for example, wholehearted living with others involves being awake to another's vulnerability with a sensitivity that moves one to affirm the wholeness of the other to continue and flourish. Living from the heart is listening to hear the discourse of positive and negative desires of our embodied selves, making it possible to hear the desires of another. When their call is heard with the heart, that hearing is total and empowering, generating authentic action. Thus interpreting human choice from the grounding end of gentle touch, compassion (awakened with passion) is viewed to be the author of expressions of ethical, intimate, caring human touch.

In contrast, an example of disembodiment reveals how this process leads to decreased awareness of self and others' vulnerability. Alienation and a lack of self-esteem and selfhood is recognized in the literature as characteristic of persons living by means of violent "taking" lives, whether it is of objects, places, or persons. To know the potential range of human action is an awesome responsibility. Griffin (1982) reminds us that "the most dangerous kind of ignorance is ignorance of myself" (p. 641). If we do not know our own capacity to wound or destroy, as well as to care and to heal, we do not know ourselves very well. We embody an inherent paradoxical human condition. Within this view, integrity of self and strength come from knowledge of the shadows as well as the healthy side of ourselves. Without this awareness, our very self is weak. Consequently, the lack of self-awareness and inevitably self-care often diminishes our vision and subsequently our motivation to care for others. More pathetic is the possibility of choosing a destructive path of life. As one becomes less reflective and more compulsive, it is easier for us to be uncritically persuaded by commands from multiple voices. We are more likely to lack discernment and quickly and blindly obey. Being disembodied from ourselves, from our own vulnerability, the possibility of authentic human choice is greatly strained, if not totally absent. To distinguish between the subtle tendencies toward one or the other extremes of vulnerability and the continuum of human touching requires more than common sense. The following extreme examples of touching can be recognized in everyday occurrences.

Commonly, withholding information from a person needing to make a decision is considered cruel and brings on undue suffering for them. Providing needed information to a person who is facing a decision before choosing options is an act that empowers that person to respond (with understanding) to the demands of the situation. Withholding such information critical for another's life does not emote from reasons of the heart; if we are awake even a little to our shared human solidarity with another, withholding would be an infliction entwined with our own human personhood and would be intolerable to us; we would recognize the infliction as self-infliction. More likely, withholding information here emotes from reasons of the disembodied mind (without heart) akin to Cartesian dualism taken to its extreme conclusions of complete separation body and soul without flux and flow. Mechanized acts to function like a clock are unfortunately made possible through indoctrination and processes of "dis-membering." Such disassociative states are tolerable because they are not "felt" as human acts of interconnection or relation with another. The reasons for such diverse directions taken in the path of life of human beings, one so destructive, the other so caring, compells me to consider other more adequate interpretations. Without clarity of vision it is not possible to understand what appears to be human choices in life. However, the question of necessary and sufficient conditions for choice to exist is prompted by the constraints and obstacles placed upon the persons in the examples used in this chapter; were they truly free to make a choice?

Roads Taken More or Less: Hermeneutic Interpretations

What were the roads taken by each participant in the above examples that made the difference in human conduct?

From the behavioral text (the actions, interactions, context, and life-world) one can interpret the torturer as one variation of a disemboded person reduced to the mechanistic neuromuscular reactions to conditioned responses (unreflected upon), trained to "go off on command." The journey toward "torture touching" from such interpretation illuminates the intentional processes of the torturer: Torture touching occurs through stimulus-response conditioning, a training of an individual similar to the training of death squads or soldiers, to react without thought of the contextual moment nor of feelings or associations that might surface in the moment by virtue of the resemblance between torturer and tortured as members of the same species (Santiago, 1990)—yes, as persons with families, memories, hopes, and dreams for the future.

The tortured person, in contrast, is usually one who has not forgotten his or her own vulnerability and has been willing to undergo the struggles (suffer with) and remain connected to others whose human vulnerability is now being intensified by torture (Reeder, 1992). By remaining embodied in spite of pain, the wounded person manifests a willingness to stay connected on the heartful journey with others for a common purpose (to end the war)! Staying on the journey in spite of torture empowers and encourages each sojourner because they have not alienated themselves from a shared identity as an embodied people; the shared discourse of a people's desires continues to be lived out with ever more conviction, empowered by the transformation of their vulnerable hearts through compassion. Clear insight and vision of a future motivates them to keep the conviction to live a dignified life, to continue to walk "the most human walk," and to be sustained over the long haul. Such an interpretation by the people themselves illuminates a clear understanding of living from the heart in solidarity with vulnerable persons. These interpretations are consistent with numerous stories told by families of the "disappeared" in El Salvador during my visitation after the Accords were signed following 13 years of civil war (Reeder, 1992).

Implications

Losing touch with oneself is like a *forgetfulness* of tender moments with oneself, with one's God, and with others. The ethical imperative for our era in the moral history of humankind (Scheler, 1974) is to reawaken reverence and respect for our embodied presence to one another and to have a certain awe about the body as the opportunity and "gracious meeting place" for the unfolding of a future together.

Nurses, among all helping professions, have a privileged position where presence and human touch are our most precious assets. Our responsibilities depend on listening as we journey along vulnerable passages through the heart. Without these existential cues, meaningful relationships with others are not possible. If compassionate caring is embarking on a vulnerable journey of passages through the heart, then awakening vulnerability is the kind of emotive education that students of nursing are in most need of learning and discerning.

The idea of education, "educare" (to care for the possibilities of life) assumes there is a future to look forward to in which to place hope. Havel (1988) writes that "hope is not prognostication. . . . and is definitely not the same thing as optimism. It is not the conviction that something will turn out well, but the certainty that something makes sense, regardless of how it turns out" (p. 20). Hope is signaled on the journey through the heart by the presence of an active imagination, creating a future out of the possibilities one envisions. Most of all, learning to live from the heart serves as a reminder that all that is strange and foreign can become familiar through sharing passages of the heart with another.

The role of the imagination and the realm of possibility indicate that learning how to live a caring life involves a sharing of our very selves, our present realities, and our dreams and hopes for the future. More than the day-to-day passages of the heart is required in addition to the conception and image of a preferred world of caring and being cared for. A pedagogical model can serve as a reminder to students of the heights and depths to which they can aspire while on the journey of caring and is a subject for yet another paper.

References

Amnesty International. (1992). *Annual report*. London: Author.

Gadow, S. (1988). Covenant without cure: Letting go and holding on in chronic illness. In J. Watson & M. Ray (Eds.), *The ethics of care and the ethics of cure: Synthesis in chronicity* (pp. 5-14). New York: National League for Nursing.

Green, M. (1988). *The dialectic of freedom*. New York: Teachers College Press.

Griffin, S. (1982). The way of all ideology. *Journal of Women in Culture and Society, 7*(3), 641-655.

Havel, V. (1988). *Letters to Olga*. New York: Alfred A. Knopf.

Reeder, F. (1992). *Personal memoirs of mercy delegation to El Salvador: August 1992*. Unpublished manuscript, University of Colorado, Denver.

Rogers, M. E. (1970). *An introduction to the theoretical basis of nursing*. Philadelphia: F. A. Davis.

Santiago, D. (1990, March 24). The aesthetics of terror, the hermeneutics of death. *America*, pp. 292-295.

Scheler, M. (1974). Ethics and the "Era of Harmonization" in A. Deeken (Ed.), *Process and permanence in ethics: Max Scheler's moral philosophy* (pp. 221-258). New York: Paulist Press.

Ward, H. (1894). *Oxford English dictionary* (p. 329). Oxford, UK: Oxford University Press.

Suggested Readings

Healey, J. (1990, Summer). *Amnesty action newsletter*. New York: Amnesty International.

Husserl, E. (1973). *Experience and judgment: Investigations of the geneology of logic*. Evanston, IL: Northwestern University Press.

Oppenheim, F. M. (Ed.). (1986). *The reasoning heart: Theological studies*. Washington, DC: Georgetown University Press.

Reeder, F. (1984). *Nursing research, holism and philosophy of science: Points of congruence between Martha E. Rogers and Edmund Husserl*. Unpublished doctoral dissertation, New York University. (University Microfilms No. 84-21,466)

Reeder, F. (1988). Grounded in self in both caring and curing. In J. Watson & M. Ray (Eds.), *The ethics of care and the ethics of cure: Synthesis in chronicity* (pp. 41-44). New York: National League for Nursing.

Richards, M. C. (1989). *Centering: Pottery, poetry and the person* (25th anniversary ed.). Middletown, CT: Wesleyan University Press.

Steindl-Rast, D. (1984). Wholeheartedness. In *Gratefulness, the heart of prayer: An approach to life in fullness*. New York: Paulist Press.

Teilhard de Chardin, P. (1978). *The heart of matter.* New York: Harcourt Brace Jovanovich.

Williams, D. D. (1981). *The spirit and the forms of love.* Lanham, NY: University Press of America.

Critical Theory for Science of Nursing Practice

HESOOK SUZIE KIM

INGER MARGRETHE HOLTER

T here has been some interest shown by nursing scholars in recent years in critical theory as nursing scientists began to question the validity of positivism and the limitations of interpretivism and hermeneutics in addressing key issues in the development of nursing knowledge (Allen, 1985, 1986; Allen, Benner, & Diekelmann, 1986; Hedin, 1986; Holter, 1988; Kendall, 1992; Ray, 1992). Such interest has pointed out the need to rethink nursing practice not only as problem-solving "work" but also as praxis in which nurses as human agents are engaged in interactions and coordination of interpersonal and personal actions. Although Kim (1994) suggests that there are four possible positions that offer specific types of explanation and knowledge regarding nursing practice— rationalist, interpretivist, mediation, and emancipation—it is the emancipation position that specifically addresses this reframing of nursing practice toward self-reflection and a movement to a newer dimension of practice. Nursing practice involves interpersonal exchanges between clients and nurses in which ideas, information, intentions, and desires about nursing care needs and nursing actions are communicated and shared. Hence the key force involved in such exchanges is mutual understanding, and the question thus is how to arrive at such mutual understanding. Critical theory offers a framework that can be applied to nursing practice for this purpose.

In this chapter, a brief historical background regarding the development of critical theory is presented, followed by an outline of the essence of the epistemology of critical theory advanced by Habermas. Habermas's theory of communicative action is then described, followed by a proposal to apply that theory in nursing practice.

Historical Background for the Development of Critical Philosophy

Critical theory has its origin in Germany in what is now referred to as the Frankfurt school. It began with the establishment of the Institute for Social Research in the 1920s as left-wing intellectuals in Germany felt a need to reappraise Marxist theory in light of what was happening in the political and economic scene in Europe and move the notion of domination beyond economic and class struggle. However, its movement went through various stages from this beginning to its most active development during the 1950s through the 1970s. When Max Horkheimer became the Institute's director in 1931 the scholars in the Institute began to develop the ideas of critical theory. Under Horkheimer's influence, the Institute became known as an interdisciplinary research center oriented toward the "restatement of Marxism in the form of a critical theory of society" (Kortian, 1980, p. 8). Besides Horkheimer, others such as Herbert Marcuse and Theodor Adorno contributed to the foundation of critical theory. However, it was Horkheimer who formulated the principal ideas. These ideas are expressed in his development of the notion of a social philosophy, the role of which is to develop criticism of positivism. Horkheimer claimed that critical theorists reject the positivistic view of science. He further claimed that the paramount importance for the development of a critical school of thought was the task of protecting human beings from false consciousness that might blind them from understanding their true interests. Thus the aim of critical theory from the very beginning has been to create a life free of all forms of unnecessary domination. Horkheimer (1976) states that "critical theory never aims simply at an increase in knowledge as such. The goal is man's emancipation from slavery" (p. 224). Horkheimer also had a strong opinion about methodology, as he believed that no one method could produce definitive results about any given object of inquiry (Held, 1980). Hence the development of critical theory also represented an attempt to formulate an alternative epistemology for social theory (Bottomore, 1984).

The criticism of positivism and the attempt to formulate an alternative epistemology and method for social research provided the fundamental principle behind the works produced at the Frankfurt school. A cross-fertilization of ideas among the members of the school also occurred along with the development of their work oriented to analyzing social conditions of domination and proposing approaches to remedy such domination. However, the individual differences among the members in interpreting and presenting the principal ideas have made a unified understanding of critical theory impossible (Held, 1980).

With the end of World War II and the movement toward a greater social and political consciousness, the Frankfurt school's intellectuals played an important role for the radical student movement throughout Europe and the United States. Through works such as Marcuse's (1964) *One Dimensional Man*, another element in critical theory emerged: "a critical attitude towards the ideological influence of science and technology as a major factor in the creation of a new technocratic-bureaucratic form of domination" (Bottomore, 1984, p. 48). Under the dominant influence of Adorno, another interrelated element emerged that criticized the culture aspect of domination. This theme had its origin in Horkheimer and Adorno's (1991) essay "Enlightenment as Mass Deception," where they, among other things, discuss the consequences of advertising.

From the beginning of the 1970s, the central ideas of critical theory were carried on more by individuals rather than as an explicitly stated part of a research program of the Frankfurt school. The dominant individual contributor and the one who has been most associated with critical theory for the past 25 years is Jürgen Habermas. Habermas restores the collaboration between philosophy and the social sciences, which over time had become replaced and dominated by philosophy.

Habermas, in objecting to the notion of "total critique" that was embedded in the existing rationality and was advocated by Adorno, Marcuse, and Horkheimer, tries to reconstruct "a more differentiated and comprehensive account of reason" (Roderick, 1986, p. 46). He thus tries to bring critical theory beyond the level of critical self-reflection to the level of a theory. Habermas presents the basis of his interpretation and presentation of critical theory in his 1971 work, *Knowledge and Human Interests*. In this work, he carries on the heritage of the Frankfurt school's tradition by a continual refinement of central criticism of positivism and by an attempt to formulate an alternative epistemology for social theory.

Habermas's Epistemology

In *Knowledge and Human Interests*, Habermas (1971) presents a new way of epistemological reflection by offering a comprehensive framework for knowledge specified into three categories. He claims that there are specific viewpoints from which we can apprehend social reality. These viewpoints represent three categories of knowledge, or cognitive interests, as Habermas calls them. They are identified as technical, practical, and emancipatory interests and are viewed as distinct but interrelated domains of knowledge. The *technical cognitive interest* focuses on technical control, with an emphasis on practical reason in dealing with objects, and thus points to the empirical-analytic sciences. The *practical cognitive interest* is oriented to understanding in social life, with an emphasis on reflective judgment and interpretive understanding, and hence points to historical-hermeneutic sciences. The *emancipatory cognitive interest* focuses on the freeing of individuals from constraints and domination, with an emphasis on critical and self-reflection for mutual understanding, and thus points to critically oriented sciences.

Through the application of empirical-analytic science, predictive knowledge is gained that leads to purposeful, rational action. Empirical-analytic knowledge is that which is embodied in the natural sciences. Within these sciences, one seeks to explain the inherent orderliness of nature in a nexus of cause and effect. By isolating objects and events into dependent and independent variables, it is possible to manipulate the environment and ensure successful action. This makes predictions possible that can expand the human power of technical control.

According to Habermas (1971), the task of the empirical-analytic sciences is the generation of technical knowledge.

In contrast to the search for empirical regularities, the historical-hermeneutic sciences constitute practical knowledge through the understanding of meaning provided by an intersubjective interpretation of social situations. This intersubjectivity allows one to comprehend the situation from the perspective and context of another, from the inside out rather than outside in, so to speak: "Access to the fact is provided by the understanding of meaning, not observation" (Habermas, 1971, p. 309). Whereas the empirical-analytic method encourages objective distance between the investigators and subjects, the hermeneutic method emphasizes the analysis of text and meaning through a subject-subject relationship more amenable to the goal of understanding meaning. The hermeneutic structure was designed to "guarantee, within cultural traditions, the possible action-orienting self-understanding between different individuals and groups" (Habermas, 1971, p. 176). Habermas (1971) argues further that in the development of knowledge of socio-cultural phenomena the researcher must penetrate the language and social context of the object.

The knowledge created from the empirical-analytic and historical-hermeneutic sciences is fundamental in arriving at a knowledge that may be necessary for social existence, but this is not sufficient, according to Habermas, to fully comprehend social phenomena. Habermas is not only critical of the monopolic claims of the empirical-analytic sciences, he is also critical of the universal claim of the historical-hermeneutic sciences. He argues that any reduction of the social sciences to the understanding of subjective meanings fails to recognize that these understandings are themselves heavily influenced by a context that can limit both the scope of the individual situation and the possibility of changing it. The hermeneutic method is thus not sufficient because it provides no critical basis for interpreting the nature of the problematic situation. Habermas stresses that the goal of systematic social sciences, such as economics, sociology, and political science, as well as the empirical-analytic sciences is to produce nomological knowledge, or lawlike knowledge. There must also be knowledge that is oriented to liberating individuals from the constraint of domination and distorted communication and allows them to be involved in the process of their own emancipation.

Habermas (1975) claims that knowledge that is created from the critically oriented sciences has a derivative status as it begins with an acknowledgment and necessity of the knowledge from the empirical-analytic and historical-hermeneutic sciences but goes beyond by reconciling them and moving toward emancipation. The emancipatory interest in this form is concerned with the power relationship between theoretical knowledge and the objective domain of practical social life, which comes into existence as a result of systematically distorted communication. Critical theory strives to go beyond the lawlike "frozen" structure of nomology and encourages a "process of reflection in the consciousness of those to whom the laws are about" (Habermas, 1971, p. 197). The goal of critical theory is to release the individual from the constraint of domination and distorted communication by creating knowledge that furthers autonomy and responsibility. Critical theory aims at bringing self-knowledge and self-reflection to an individual whose perception of a situation is clouded by values imposed by society. That individual is, in general, led to believe that the self-perception is a function of the self's own true condition rather than a condition imposed by social codes. Social institutions can be repressive, thwarting the individual in the pursuit of true desires by creating a false consciousness and a constrained existence. The individual interprets the social institution's values as personal ones in a form of self-imposed coercion. Thus critical theory initiates a "process of self-enlightenment of socialized individuals about what they would want if they knew what they could want" (Habermas, cited in Geuss, 1981, p. 83). By having an orientation built from the three categories of knowledge, a viewpoint is established that promotes autonomy and responsibility and from which communication can be "developed into nonauthoritarian and universal dialogue" (Habermas, 1971, p. 314).

Habermas's work in *Knowledge and Human Interest* has been the center of extensive criticism and discussion to which he has continuously responded. The outcome of this answering process "of rejecting what is no longer defensible, preserving what he still deems valid, and moving beyond earlier formulations to new frontiers" (Bernstein, 1985, p. 15) has led to a substantial revision and expansion of Habermas's thinking, which has resulted in a shift in a grounding of critical theory from the epistemological sphere to the development of a theory that is oriented to a proactive posture regarding emancipation. However, Habermas develops this theory within the epistemological arguments posed in his *Knowledge and Human Interests.* The overall goal of critical theory is to shape a life free of all forms of unnecessary domination. This life is based on emancipation and requires both enlightenment and action. Hence Habermas considers communicative action as the foundation as a way of attaining this goal.

Habermas's Theory of Communicative Action

The development of the concepts that form the theory of communicative action can be discerned throughout Habermas's various publications and books. The primary focus of the following presentation is on explicating the basic concepts of the theory of communicative action and outlining the major tenets of the theory from Habermas's various writings. For Habermas, the concept of communicative action refers to the interaction of at least two persons who are capable of speech and action. The participants seek to achieve an understanding about the situation of action and their plans of action by arriving at an agreement so that their future actions may be coordinated.

In a broader framework in his consideration of social actions, Habermas considers communicative action and strategic action the major analytic aspects of social actions: Communicative action is oriented to reaching an interpersonal understanding and as action where the participants are not primarily interested in attaining their own individual successes but in arriving at their individual goals through mutual understanding and harmonious interpretations of what are at stake, whereas strategic action is oriented to individual successes and as "a reciprocal influencing of one another by opponents acting in a purposive-rational manner" (Habermas, 1984a, p. 286). Hence he holds that any social action can be analytically described in both ways.

Two major concepts undergird Habermas's theory of communicative action: communicative competence and ideal speech situation. Communicative competence refers to competence in speech and symbolic interaction as well as linguistic competence. To have communicative competence means the mastery of what he calls an ideal speech situation. Habermas (1984a) presents the four types of speech acts that he claims represent a general classification of speech acts necessary for an ideal speech situation:

1. *Constative* speech acts in which the true value of utterances is the key
2. *Representative* speech acts in which the self-representation of the speaker is made
3. *Regulative* speech acts in which the normative status of rules is expressed
4. *Communicative* speech acts that serve to express different aspects of the very purpose of speech

Habermas's theory of communicative action based on the above conceptualizations stems from his ideas about comprehensive rationality that is the foundation for his epistemology and encompasses the theory of argumentation that is founded upon communicative rationality. His point of departure for the development of the concept of communicative rationality is the assumption that there is a close relationship between knowledge and rationality. He further claims that rationality concerns how a person acquires and uses knowledge, and is reflected in human actions. Habermas (1984a) proposes a comprehensive concept of rationality claiming that rationality from a realist perspective in which actions "basically have the character of goal-directed, feedback-controlled interventions" is too narrow to capture the rationality inherent in a communicative practice (p. 12). His idea is that a comprehensive concept of communicative rationality can be developed from merging the realist's goal-directed action perspective with the phenomenologist's meaningful action perspective. He expands this internal relationship to also include what he calls normative regulative action and expressive self-reflections. The communicative rationality thus becomes the basis for "the central experience of the unconstrained, unifying, consensus-bringing force of argumentative speech, in which different participants overcome their merely subjective views and, owing to the mutuality of rationally motivated conviction, assure themselves of both the unity of the objective world and the intersubjectivity of their lifeworld" (p. 10).

Such rationality thus is inherent in communicative practice and forms the ground for criticizable validity claims embedded in speech acts that are exchanged. Habermas hence specifies the normative dimension on what it means to be involved in a speech act by proposing the thesis that "anyone acting communicatively must, in performing any speech action, raise universal validity claims and suppose that they can be vindicated" (p. 2). Because communicative action, according to Habermas, is oriented to consensus and understanding among participants as a means to coordinate their plans of action, agreement among the interactive participants on validity claims entrenched within speech acts is the key to intersubjective understanding and coordination of actions.

He specifies four different validity claims underlying speech acts for reaching intersubjective understanding: *truth, rightness, truthfulness,* and *comprehensibility*. The truth validity claim is contained in the constative speech acts. The speaker must have the intention of communicating a true or correct existential proposition so that the hearer can share the knowledge of the speaker in the sense that there is an agreement about the utterance's propositional truth. The validity claim of rightness is contained in the regulative speech acts. The speech act performed must be judged to be right normatively within the context of action. Hence the utterance is evaluated by the hearer for its rightness in the norma- tive sense and for legitimating the intersubjective relations expressed in the situation. The validity claim of truthfulness is contained in the representative speech acts. The expression is truthful expression of one's beliefs, intentions, feelings, and desires to suggest credibility and sincerity. The comprehensibility validity claim is contained in the com- municative speech acts. The expression is comprehensible for mutually agreeable interpretations in that the speaker must choose a compre- hensible expression so that the speaker and the hearer can understand one another. These four validity claims embedded in speech acts provide for the intersubjective commonality of a communicatively achieved agreement at the levels of shared propositional knowledge, normative accord, mutual trust in subjective sincerity, and mutual comprehension (Habermas, 1979, 1984a).

If the listener doubts any of the claims conveyed by the speaker, then both can explicitly discuss the validity of the validity claims. Habermas (1984a) proposes a theory of argumentation as a way that such discus- sions should take place. Argumentation thus is conceptualized as "that type of speech in which participants thematize contested validity claims and attempt to vindicate or criticize them through arguments" (p. 18). Habermas presents five different modes of argumentation in which contested validity claims can be vindicated or criticized. In an argumentation in the form of a *theoretical discourse*, controversial truth claims are contested by the hearer to which the responses would take the form of logical validation and explanations. In an argumentation in the form of a *practical discourse*, the rightness claims are made thematic by the hearer to which justification is the method of response. In an argumentation in the form of an *aesthetic criticism*, the adequacy of value standards is thematized. Because the adequacy of value standards can only be subjected to argumentation in relation to its intrasubjective validity rather than the universal one, the criticism must center around the truthfulness and sincerity of an expression to which self-representation is the method of response. In an argumentation in the form of a *therapeutic critique*, the expressions of the speaker's own desires and feelings are contested as the hearer perceives them to be systematically self-deceptive. Habermas uses the notion of therapeutic critique from Freud's psychoanalytic perspective and does not use this form of argumentation in illustrating his theory, especially in his later works. It appears that he acknowledges the affinity of this form of argumentation with aesthetic criticism. Self-deception is addressed through self-reflection. In an argumentation in the form of an *explicative discourse*, the comprehensibility claims are contested by the hearer to which an interpretation is a mode of response. Habermas later prefers to regard comprehensibility as a preparatory condition rather than a validity claim as it does not raise a criticizable claim about objective, social, and subjective reality (Ingram, 1987, p. 201). By participating in argumentation a person can either acknowledge or ignore the force of the reasons represented in the argument. However, a mutual interpersonal understanding is only possible with participation in argumentation as it arises out of communicative practice among people.

Habermas not only expands his characterizations of an ideal speech situation through the presentation of the validity claims contained in the different speech acts, but he also derives from the four speech acts the symmetric and reciprocity conditions for an ideal speech situation to take place. Symmetric conditions provide for equal chances for all participants to employ communicative speech acts and to put forward the validity claims. Reciprocity conditions provide for equal chances of expressing one's views, feelings, and wishes and equal chances to resist, to allow and forbid, to make and retract a promise, to be accountable, and to owe an explanation (Habermas, 1984b, p. 177-178). When such conditions are not assured, the participants would not be able to engage freely in different forms of argumentation for attaining mutual understanding of their exchanges. Therefore, communicative practice cannot be sustained to produce mutual understanding of goals and

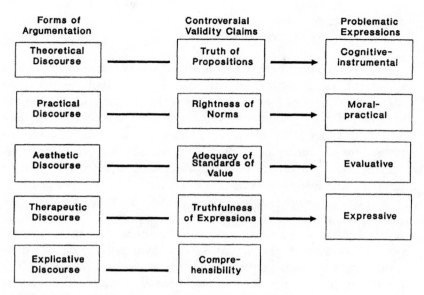

FIGURE 15.1. Habermas's theory of argumentation

coordination of actions, and the interpersonal exchanges may contain the elements of domination. Figure 15.1 shows the major aspects of Habermas's theory of argumentation as described henceforth.

Participants in social action may be engaged in strategic actions with openness about the specific goals in which disputes regarding the validity claims are irrelevant as participants are engaged in "a reciprocal influencing of one another by opponents acting in a purposive-rational manner" (Habermas, 1984a, p. 286). However, there are strategic actions in which the goals are concealed either consciously or unconsciously. Habermas (1984a) calls these (a) manipulation containing conscious deception and (b) systematically distorted communication in which there is unconscious deception. Deetz (1992) claims that systematically distorted communication is rather common and that it can be pathological when it "(1) endangers the survival of the human and other species by limiting important adaptations to a changing environment, (2) violates normative standards already freely shared by members of the community, and (3) poses arbitrary limits on the development of individualization and the realization of collective goods" (p. 177).

Application to Nursing:
Toward a Theory for Nursing Practice

Kim (1994) claims that nursing must develop practice theories that are applicable in designing practitioners' actions in their relationships with clients as nursing practice involves working with and attending to clients as communicative agents in interactive contexts. Nursing practice with this focus then can be considered human-to-human service with a view of clients not as clinical events but as experiencing and communicating persons. Both clients and practitioners are engaged in interactive and intertwined human activities where practice is a part of continuous human engagement. From this orientation a theory of nursing practice expanding on Habermas's theory of communicative action is developed as a theoretical framework on which nurses' actions, especially as a form of social action, are explained and prescriptive nursing practice is formulated. This theory offers a way of understanding nurses' engagement in practice as an agent of human action and is a generalized action theory of nursing practice in which nurses' "talk" is conceptualized as a medium through which nursing's instrumental actions directed toward clients are processed and eventuated in practice.

A theory of nursing practice with a focus on nurses' communicative action is developed as a way of addressing nursing's emancipatory cognitive interest. The social climate that prevails in the current practice of nursing indicates an existence of oppression of different client groups and concentration of power in dominant groups. Furthermore, the institutions of the health care system tend to function within the culture of economic and rational decision making. Although a great stride has taken place to empower consumers of health care, patients still perceive their roles as passive and dependent (Kim et al., 1993). True empowerment of clients of nursing care then can come about through the processes in which mutual understanding about the health care processes is attained.

The theory proposes four forms of rational prescriptions—*theoretical, practical, aesthetic,* and *explicative discourses*—for nurses' communicative action as a way of avoiding strategic communication that tends to be oriented to unilateral success. While some nursing actions are necessarily strategic, especially when the goals of action are manifestly understood both by the nurse and client on the purposive-rational grounds, most nursing actions may become ineffective or inefficient when they are not based on a mutual understanding concerning their goals. By applying theoretical, practice, aesthetic, and explicative discourses nurses can provide opportunities for arriving at mutual understanding with clients so that coordinated nursing actions may eventuate in the situation of patient care. Hence this is a *normative* communicative action theory of nursing practice through which prescriptive nursing approaches to patients can be designed.

An application of these five forms of argumentation in nursing practice then involves the nurse *questioning* the validity claims embedded in the client's utterances or *responding* to the client's criticism about the nurse's claims in order to provide communicative rationality. Let us assume that a patient expresses the following statement to a nurse when the nurse asked the patient to ambulate on the second postoperative day:

I cannot go for a walk. I am afraid that my gut will fall out if I walk.

The nurse then can contest the truth claim of these statements (theoretical discourse):

Your gut will not fall out even if you walked since it is very well secured.

Or the nurse may contest the rightness claim of these statements (practical discourse):

All patients with the kind of operation you had are required to ambulate as soon as possible.

Or the nurse may question the truthfulness of these statements (aesthetic discourse):

Are you sure you are refusing because you are afraid?

The application of explicative discourse for the comprehensibility claim is embedded in the total exchange, as the fundamental premise for the exchange to take place is that both the nurse and client use language and speech forms that are comprehensible. The nurse must especially avoid using professional and technical language in her communication.

Application of the theory of communicative action as illustrated and adopted to nursing practice situation will facilitate emancipation of clients. However, the context of nursing practice also must be emancipatory for the nurses to apply such a theory. Application of the theory of argumentation in situations of nursing practice is appropriate when there is misunderstanding of meanings, differences in interpretation of meanings, or disparity in views or when participants are not honest in their expression of feelings and actions. Such instances will produce distortions in communication, a lack of a mutual understanding about goals, and impede learning and personal growth. Therefore, it is essential that the process of argumentation be applied with the goal of attaining mutual understanding and emancipation of participants, that is, both nurses and clients, from constraints and biases.

Summary

By proposing the theory of communicative action, Habermas brought forward the level of exposition in critical theory to a more concrete level. Furthermore, his critical theory transcends the dead-end nature of self-centered reflection of both the early critical theorists and the postmodernists and moves toward conscious reconstruction and change from the level of individual communication to the social level. Applicability of critical theory and the theory of communicative action to nursing is evident when we view nursing practice as involving collaboration and mutual process between the nurse and client and also necessitating the empowerment of clients and enhancement of clients' lot within the health care system.

References

Allen, D. (1985). Nursing research and social control: Alternative models of science that emphasize understanding and emancipation. *Image, 12*(2), 58-64.

Allen, D. (1986). Using philosophical and historical methodologies to understand the concept of health. In P. Chinn (Ed.), *Nursing research methodology: Issues and implementation* (pp. 157-164). Rockville, MD: Aspen Systems.

Allen, D., Benner, P., & Diekelmann, N. (1986). Three paradigms for nursing research: Methodological implications. In P. Chinn (Ed.), *Nursing research methodology: Issues and implementation* (pp. 23-38). Rockville, MD: Aspen Systems.

Bernstein, R. (1985). *Habermas and modernity*. Cambridge: MIT Press.

Bottomore, T. (1984). *The Frankfurt school*. Chichester: Ellis Horwood Limited.

Deetz, S. (1992). *Democracy in an age of corporate colonization*. Albany: State University of New York Press.

Geuss, R. (1981). *The idea of critical theory: Habermas and the Frankfurt school.* Cambridge: Cambridge University Press.

Habermas, J. (1971). *Knowledge and human interests.* Boston: Beacon.

Habermas, J. (1975). A postscript to knowledge and human interest. *Philosophy of the Social Sciences, 2,* 157-189.

Habermas, J. (1979). Communication and the evolution of society. Boston: Beacon.

Habermas, J. (1984a). *The theory of communicative action: Volume 1.* Boston: Beacon.

Habermas, J. (1984b). *Vorstudien und Erganzungen zur Theorie des 1 kommunikative Handelns [Preliminary studies and supplements to the theory of commuicative action].* Frankfurt: Suhrkamp.

Hedin, B. (1986). Nursing, education, and emancipation: Applying the critical theoretical approach to nursing research. In P. Chinn (Ed.), *Nursing research methodology: Issues and implementation* (pp. 133-156). Rockville, MD: Aspen Systems.

Held, D. (1980). *Introduction to critical theory: Horkheimer to Habermas.* Berkeley: University of California Press.

Holter, I. M. (1988). Critical theory: A foundation for the development of nursing theories. *Scholarly Inquiry for Nursing Practice: An International Journal, 2,* 223-232.

Horkheimer, M. (1976). Traditional and critical theory. In P. Connerton (Ed.), *Critical sociology* (pp. 224-227). Harmondsworth: Penguin.

Horkheimer, M., & Adorno, T. (1991). Enlightment as mass deception. In T. W. Adorno & J. M. Bernstein (Eds.), *The culture industry: Selected essays on mass culture* (pp. 68-88). New York: Routledge.

Ingram, D. (1987). *Habermas and the dialectic of reason.* New Haven, CT: Yale University Press.

Kendall, J. (1992). Fighting back: Promoting emancipatory nursing actions. *Advances in Nursing Science, 15,* 1-15.

Kim, H. S. (1994). Practice theories in nursing and a science of nursing practice. *Scholarly Inquiry for Nursing Practice: An International Journal, 8,* 123-137.

Kim, H. S., Holter, I. M., Lorensen, M., Inayoshi, M., Shimaguchi, S., Shimazaki-Ryder, R., Kawaguchi, Y., Hori, R., Takezaki, K., Leino-Kilpi, H., & Munkki-Utunen, M. (1993). Patient-nurse collaboration: A comparison of patients' and nurses' attitudes in Japan, Norway, Finland and USA. *International Journal of Nursing Studies,* (30), 387-401.

Kortian, G. (1980). *Metacritique: The philosophical argument of Jürgen Habermas.* Cambridge: University of Cambridge Press.

Marcuse, H. (1964). *One-dimensional man.* Boston: Beacon.

Ray, M. (1992). Critical theory as a framework to enhance nursing science. *Nursing Science Quarterly, 5,* 98-100.

Roderick, R. (1986). *Habermas and the foundation of critical theory.* New York: St. Martin's.

Suggested Readings

Bernstein, R. (1983). *Beyond objectivism and relativism.* Philadelphia: University of Pennsylvania Press.

Habermas, J. (1973). *Theory and practice.* Boston: Beacon.

Habermas, J. (1988). *On the logic of the social sciences.* Cambridge: Polity.

16

Methodology for Critical Theory

Critical Action Research

INGER MARGRETHE HOLTER

HESOOK SUZIE KIM

Research methodology that adopts critical theory as the basis for knowledge development has neither been specifically advanced by Habermas nor by researchers in social sciences, although there has been a great deal of debates about appropriateness and application of various methods. The debate center around the necessity and development of a "new" method of inquiry logically appropriate with the foundational premises of critical theory.

Fischer (1985), in search of a methodology of critical theory for public policy analysis, suggests "a critical evaluation" as a method of examining both the empirical and normative assumptions behind a specific policy. His method of critical evaluation encompasses four phases that interrelate two fundamental levels of evaluation: the first-order discourse consisting of verification and validation and the second-order discourse composed of vindication and rational social choice. Therefore, his method is not only oriented to evaluating the empirical elements but also the evaluation of normative assumptions undergirding a specific social policy. However, this method focuses on examination of social policy as praxis rather than social action. Hence his approach is founded on Habermas's epistemology of critical sciences rather than specifically on Habermas's communicative action and the theory of argumentation. Morrow (1991) with a somewhat different stance argues for a necessity of expanding the concept of methodology that incorporates "the full ranges of logical, empirical and normative arguments which make up the process of scientific argumentation" (p. 224). He further indicates that conventional and alternative methodological approaches should be justified and criticized in terms of their relations to critical social science as any approach must be embedded in a particular context of inquiry and argumentation. In this sense, Morrow does not offer a specific critical theory methodology but suggests that any methodology must be subjected to self-criticism from a comprehensive critical theory of methodology. He uses the theory of argumentation as the way of carrying out such self-criticism regarding methodology used in a program of research.

Deetz (1985), in reviewing the work in cultural research in organization, found that although there has been some interest in the direction of research toward the critical perspective there is a lack of methodological development to deal with the critical perspective. However, Deetz suggests that "participative research" holds a promise for addressing the organizational issues related to distorted communication arising from domination.

In a similar manner, Comstock (1982) argues that it is not appropriate to just apply "the investigative logic developed by the positive social sciences to new topics and expect to develop a truly critical social science" (p. 371). He considers research in critical theory as starting with "the life problems of definite and particular social agents who may be individuals, groups, or classes that are oppressed by and alienated from social processes they maintain or create but do not control" (p. 378). Comstock thus outlines seven steps of critical research method:

1. Identification of specific social agent(s) who are interested in change of practice and able to participate in research

2. Development of a hermeneutic understanding of participants' meanings of the situation

3. Empirical analyses of social structures and processes of the context

4. Construction of integrated understanding through the dialectics of individual interpretations and meanings within a specific context with its history, structures, and processes

5. Enlightenment of participants of their oppression by identifying the elements of truth in an ideology from the context of falsity

6. Emancipatory education of participants in which participants themselves develop new understandings and actions

7. Participation in critical education that is a theoretically grounded program of action for the elimination of further social injustice

These suggestions and arguments by various authors interpret Habermas's positions regarding methodology with somewhat different foci; furthermore, their proposals tend to fall short of specificity in terms of research strategies. Whereas most authors seem to be interested in espousing general approaches for critical theory methodology, Comstock (1982) offers a set of specific guidelines for developing a critical method of research. In the following sections, we present Habermas's ideas about critical theory methodology and offer a *critical action research* as a method of inquiry that builds on the shared assumptions in critical theory and in action research. Application of critical action research in nursing is discussed in the concluding section.

Habermas's Proposal

In defending his thesis that a critical theory of society faces rationality on both the metatheoretical and methodological level (Habermas, 1984, pp. 7, 75), Habermas has explicated a foundation for a methodology consistent with his metatheory. He claims that there is an interdependence between the basic concepts of action and the methodology of understanding social science. Habermas (1984) proposes the thesis that a researcher can only interpret communicative action rationally. The way to gain access to real data of communicative action is through rational interpretation. This means that to understand the different speech acts and the validity claims contained in each of them, the researcher has to understand the reasons with which persons would defend their validity claims. However, the researcher cannot present reasons without making judgments about them:

> Reasons are of such a nature that they cannot be described in the attitude of a third person, that is, without reactions of affirmation or negation or abstention. . . . An interpreter cannot, therefore, interpret expression connected through criticizable validity claims with a potential of reasons without taking a position on them. And he cannot take a position without applying his own standards of judgment. (pp. 115-116)

Thus the researcher in making interpretation of reasons needs to assume the role of a virtual participant. Habermas (1984) describes this role as an interpreter who goes into the research situation without one's own aims of change or action but is only interested in gaining an understanding of the meanings of the actual situation through the judgments of validity claims. The success of the interaction between the researcher and the subjects of research will depend on a process of common interpretation "in which the participants come to a common definition of the situation within the reference system of the three worlds" (p. 119). However, a precondition for this process is that the people involved are capable of mutual criticism and that the situation allows for reciprocity and symmetry among participants. Collaboration built on the conditions of symmetry and reciprocity thus occurs as a mutual learning process for both the researcher and the practitioner. Deetz (1992) describes this learning process:

> Such a learning process, however, is not of putting people in touch with themselves or learning to articulate their insides clearly, but one that reopens engagement in the development of differentiated feelings and discursive possibilities, to participate in the affective and expressive development of self and others. (p. 176)

In being a virtual participant the researcher brings his or her own preunderstanding to the situation. Habermas builds on the work of Gadamer's hermeneutics to support this assumption. Gadamer claims that all understanding inevitably involves some prejudice (Bernstein, 1983). How the researcher's prejudice works becomes clear in Gadamer's understanding of the hermeneutical circle. Gadamer claims that the researcher is not separated from his or her prejudgments and/or prejudices. It is because the researcher has this preunderstanding that the "things themselves" can be understood. Thus there is no difference between understanding and interpretation as all understanding involves interpretation and all interpretation involves understanding. As such there is no correct interpretation. This does not mean that the individual interpretation is arbitrary or distortive. The universal criteria of honesty, openness, and precision in research is not to be violated, but the understanding will be different in relation to a person's self-understanding and the different questions which are to be asked (Bernstein, 1983).

Although accepting Gadamer's assumption about the involvement of a researcher's preunderstanding in an interpretation, Habermas (1984) is critical of the one-sidedness of Gadamer's interpretative understanding and the lack of a critical means of penetrating a given context:

> We not only admit the possibility that the interpretandum may be exemplar *for us*, that we may learn something from it; we also take into account the possibility that the author could learn *from us*. . . Processes of reaching understanding are aimed at a consensus that depends on the intersubjective recognition of validity claims; and these claims can be reciprocally raised and fundamentally criticized by the participants in the communication. (pp. 134, 136, emphases in original)

Habermas indicates that the twofold goal inherent in his metatheory has to be built into the methodology, in that the researcher not only gain interpretations from the hermeneutic sense but also reach beyond the interpretation to the level of emancipation. Thus in becoming a virtual participant the researcher must also assume the role of a change agent. This role becomes clearer when Habermas points out that the same structure for reaching an understanding also provides the "critical means to penetrate a given context . . . to push beyond a de facto established consensus" (p. 120). He claims that the researcher can bring into play those elements that are outside the actual situation and systematically apply them to the particulars.

Habermas (1984) thus espouses three key elements for critical theory methodology:

1. The researcher becomes a virtual participant in order to arrive at interpretation and understanding.

2. The researcher and participants must be involved in mutual criticism for identifying problems and developing approaches.

3. The researcher must assume the role of change agent.

These elements point to moving beyond the purely positivistic, objective stance. Habermas points out that in a communicative mode of action the requirement of objectivity is satisfied when the participants and the researcher are able to mobilize a comprehensive rationality from the objective, social and subjective worlds in reaching understanding based on the intersubjective recognition of the truth, rightness, and truthfulness claims. Habermas claims that for this requirement of objectivity to be satisfied it "would have to be shown to be universally valid in a specific sense" (p. 137). The critical theory methodology also moves beyond the interpretative design of the historical-hermeneutic methodology that is basically oriented to understanding. As the Habermas's ideas align with the basic premises underlying action research, an action research methodology founded upon critical theory is proposed in the next section.

Critical Action Research

Action research as a method of inquiry can be traced to Kurt Lewin who was involved in research to help social workers with their problems in practice (Lewin, 1947a, 1947b). Tracing the development of the different approaches of action research is in a way like following the ontological and epistemological movements that have taken place in the social and behavioral sciences in the past 50 years. One reason is that Lewin's sudden death never gave him the opportunity to clearly outline his view of philosophy of science regarding action research. Therefore, there is no answer to the question "What is Lewin's philosophical and theoretical approach to action research?" and no simple answer to the question "What is action research?" (Peters & Robinson, 1984). Although Lewin's view of social science was more in line with the hermeneutic philosophy of science reflected in his gestaltian perspective (Marrow, 1969), his writing on action research, which is very limited, is more in line with the principles of science outlined in the natural science. As recalled by Lewin's colleague, Cartwright (1978), Lewin was concerned with a fundamental flaw in his theoretical system.

> One night just shortly before his death, when he came to my house in a state of great excitement to tell me that he had just had a brilliant insight which made him see, as he put it, that "Freud was wrong and Marx was right." And he was almost euphoric when he said that this meant that he would have to make a fundamental revision in his entire theoretical approach. I still remember how surprised I was that anyone could be so pleased upon discovering a basic flaw in his own work. (p. 178)

Lewin thus left the scientific community with an ambiguous heritage that is reflected in the literature on action research in general as well as in nursing. The majority of action research conducted has been within the methodological frame of the natural sciences. The rise of the historical-hermeneutic sciences and lately also the critical social sciences have led to a development of approaches in action research that might be more in line with Lewin's last vision of revising his theoretical approach to action research than his written work (Argyris, 1980; Argyris, Putnam, & McLain Smith, 1985; Carr & Kemmis, 1986; Gustavsen, 1985; Levin, 1993).

Whereas the original concepts and method were developed within the context of social psychiatry, action research is today applied in many disciplines. There is now a variety of action research using different research designs and methods (Elden & Chrisholm, 1993; Reason, 1988; Whyte, 1991). Holter and Schwartz-Barcott (1993) outline three different approaches on which researchers have based their designs and methods in applying action research. These are the technical, the mutual, and the enhancement approaches, which respectively are founded in the natural, historical-hermeneutic, and critical social sciences. Holter and Schwartz-Barcott also outline four general features of action research as they were originally intended by its major founder, Kurt Lewin. They are (a) collaboration between researcher and practitioner, (b) identification of a practical problem, (c) change in practice, and (d) development of theory. As such, action research aims at producing new knowledge that contributes both to solving practical immediate problems and to generating knowledge (Elden & Chisholm, 1993).

Critical action research hence adopts these four features and specifies them to be congruent with the premises of critical theory.

RESEARCHER-PRACTITIONER COLLABORATION

In critical action research, there has to be collaboration between the researcher and practitioner(s) at every step of the process. Reciprocity and symmetry between the researcher and the practitioner(s) and among the practitioners themselves need to be assured to have true collaboration. Collaboration can occur in the forms of mutual criticism and self-reflection; thus it is a process involving understanding, critique, and learning.

PROBLEM IDENTIFICATION

Problem identification in critical action research involves systematic difficulties in practice. For the researcher to be a virtual participant in the setting and become involved in problem identification, he or she must develop an interpretive understanding of the context as well as the meanings held by individual practitioners in the situation. The researcher uses both empirical and hermeneutic methods to gain such insights. Total understanding of the situation is arrived at through mutual participation between the researcher and the practitioner(s). The researcher's interpretation then makes up one segment of the partite aspect of total understanding of the situation. Practitioners who are entrenched in the practical settings and have experience in how things work in the actual situation also bring their individual knowledge into the process of formulating a comprehensive understanding. In discussing individuals' interpretations of the situation, both the researcher and the practitioner(s) must assure comprehensibility of expression, normative acceptance, and truthfulness in their intentions.

As the comprehensive understanding of the situation occurs, the researcher and the practitioner(s) can begin identifying and coming to an agreement about the nature of the problems or difficulties that require change. From Habermas's perspective of critical theory, the parties involved in critical action research may not move forward from this step if any one of the participants considers the difficulties or problems only from the point of unilateral goal orientation.

INSTITUTION OF
CHANGE IN PRACTICE

The strategies for change in practice will depend on the outcome of the problem identification phase. The collaborative process that occurs in defining the practical problem(s) results in what Elden and Levin (1991) call a "local theory." Elden and Levin claim that the generation of a local theory is empowering in itself "because those who create it learn why things are as they are, and this naturally leads to ideas about change" (p. 138). The strategies for change thus emerge from the local theory. Strategies can be structural or technical as well as behavioral in nature. In critical action research, the strategies will be tested immediately and evaluated in situ so that a new or improved local theory may emerge.

The emancipatory nature of the change process gives the participants deeper understanding of their situations and may produce a more permanent impact. This is in contrast to many changes that get introduced without the involvement of practitioners, which although seeming at first to produce positive results tend to be highly superficial and overly dependent on the enthusiasm and involvement of a few key individuals.

DEVELOPMENT OF
NEW KNOWLEDGE

Through the collaborative process tacit practical knowledge is made explicit. Based on the uncovering of historical forces, economic, material, and personal conditions, a comprehensive understanding of the situation emerges. This is an enlightened knowledge that can help empower and free others from repressive, thwarting situations than merely those participating in the research. Knowledge gained from critical action research then can be used to gain generalized understanding about social conditions and praxis. Because the knowledge gained from this research is process-oriented rather than substance-oriented knowledge, it adds to the foundation upon which comprehensive understandings about the workings in practice and human actions are based.

New knowledge emerges about the action research process itself. That is, being engaged in the process of critical action research not only produces learning in the participants but also sensitivities and insights into the workings of the participative research process.

Nursing Applications

Nursing scholars have recently shown an increased interest in action research (Armitage, Champney-Smith, & Andrews, 1991; Degerhammar & Wade, 1991; Holter & Schwartz-Barcott, 1993; Lauri, 1990; McCaugherty, 1991a, 1991b; Nolan & Grant, 1993; Sheehan, 1990; Smith, 1986; Webb, 1989). The classical action research design based on the natural science approach is found in the majority of studies conducted in nursing (Holter & Schwartz-Barcott, 1993). The increasing varieties of new designs and methods in applying action research in other disciplines is yet to come in nursing. One approach to action research that is not reported in the nursing literature is the one based on the critical social sciences.

Kim (1987) outlines nursing knowledge into four domains:

1. The client domain knowledge pertaining to phenomena in the client
2. The client-nurse domain knowledge focusing on the interactive, interpersonal phenomena between the client and nurse
3. The practice domain knowledge pertaining to phenomena particular to nurses who are engaged in delivering nursing care
4. The environment domain knowledge dealing with relevant environmental and contextual phenomena

Critical theory understanding is especially relevant to both the client-nurse and practice domains. The critical action research method can thus be applied to study and produce change regarding the client-nurse relationships and the nurses' practice.

The client-nurse communications conceptualized from the critical theory perspective may point to distortions, misunderstandings, and oppression that exist in the situations of patient care. Critical action research then can be applied to illuminate such difficulties and produce changes in interactive patterns in that empowerment of both the clients and nurses may occur. Because communication is a medium through which other instrumental nursing actions are delivered, eliminating distortions and misunderstandings is critical for ensuring participative decision-making and allowing clients' self-determination. Viewing the phenomena in the nursing's practice domain from the emancipation position, Kim (1994) points to appropriateness of the application of Habermas's critical theory and critical action research as a form for studying nursing actions. Nurses' everyday practice may be entrenched within the conflicting nature of social reality of the environment of nursing practice, such as competition, role conflict, routinization, or administrative structure. Breaking away from such entrenchment involves reflection on practice and possibilities for innovative practice that is the essence specified in critical action research. This mode of change encompasses the possibilities for an enhancement of professional nursing practice.

Critical action research is a challenge for nurse researchers who are interested in bridging the gap between theory, research, and practice by empowering clients and nurses and by introducing changes in actual practice. This mode of research provides opportunities for understanding the true interests of clients and nurses, and the opportunities to create health care experiences that are free from domination. Critical action research is a practice-oriented research that occurs directly within the practice arena and contributes to the already existing research traditions in nursing.

References

Argyris, C. (1980). *Inner contradictions of rigorous research*. New York: Academic Press.

Argyris, C., Putnam, R., & McLain Smith, D. (1985). *Action science*. London: Jossey-Bass.

Armitage, P., Champney-Smith, J., & Andrews, K. (1991). Primary nursing and the role of the nurse preceptor in changing long-term mental health care: An evaluation. *Journal of Advanced Nursing, 16*, 413-422.

Bernstein, R. (1983). *Beyond objectivism and relativism*. Philadelphia: University of Pennsylvania Press.

Carr, W., & Kemmis, S. (1986). *Becoming critical: Education, knowledge and action research*. London: Falmer.

Cartwright, D.(1978). Theory and practice. *Journal of Social Issues, 34*, 168-180.

Comstock, D. (1982). A method for critical research. In E. Bredo & W. Feinberg (Eds.), *Knowledge and values in social and educational research* (pp. 370-390). Philadelphia: Temple University Press.

Deetz, S. (1985). Critical-cultural research: New sensibilities and old realities. *Journal of Management, 11,* 121-136.

Deetz, S. (1992). *Democracy in an age of corporate colonization.* Albany: State University of New York Press.

Degerhammar, M., & Wade, B. (1991). The introduction of a new system of care delivery into a surgical ward in Sweden. *International Journal of Nursing Studies, 28,* 325-336.

Elden, M., & Chisholm, R. (1993). Emerging varieties of action research: Introduction to the special issue. *Human Relations, 46,* 121-141.

Elden, M., & Levin, M. (1991). Cogenerative learning. In W. F. Whyte (Ed.), *Participatory action research* (pp. 127-142). Newbury Park, CA: Sage.

Fischer, F. (1985). Critical evaluation of public policy: A methodological case study. In J. Forester (Ed.), *Critical theory and public life* (pp. 231-257). Cambridge: MIT Press.

Gustavsen, B. (1985). Workplace reform and democratic dialogue. *Economic and Industrial Democracy, 6,* 461-479.

Habermas, J. (1984). *The theory of communicative action: Volume 1.* Boston: Beacon.

Holter, I. M., & Schwartz-Barcott, D. (1993). Action research : What is it? How has it been used in nursing research and how can it be used in nursing research? *Journal of Advanced Nursing, 18,* 298-304.

Kim, H. S. (1987). Structuring the nursing knowledge system: A typology of four domains. *Scholarly Inquiry for Nursing Practice: An International Journal, 1,* 99-110.

Kim, H. S. (1994). Practice theories in nursing and a science of nursing practice. *Scholarly Inquiry for Nursing Practice: An International Journal, 8,* 123-137.

Lauri, S. (1990). The teaching of decision-making process to nurses working in hospital. *Scandinavian Journal of Caring Science, 4,* 63-68.

Levin, M. (1993). Creating network for rural economic development in Norway. *Human Relations, 46,* 193-217.

Lewin, K. (1947a). Frontiers in group dynamics: I. Concept, method and reality in social science: Social equilibria. *Human Relations, 1,* 5-40.

Lewin, K. (1947b). Frontiers in group dynamics: II. Channels of group life: Social planning and action research. *Human Relations, 1,* 143-154.

Marrow, A. (1969). *The practical theorist: The life and work of Kurt Lewin.* New York: Basic Books.

McCaugherty, D. (1991a). The use of a teaching model to promote reflection and the experiential integration of theory and practice in first-year student nurses: An action research study. *Journal of Advanced Nursing, 16,* 534-543.

McCaugherty, D. (1991b). The theory-practice gap in nursing education: Its causes and possible solutions. Findings from an action research study. *Journal of Advanced Nursing, 16,* 1055-1061.

Morrow, R. (1991). Toward a critical theory of methodology: Habermas and the theory of argumentation. *Current Perspectives in Social Theory, 11,* 197-228.

Nolan, M., & Grant, G. (1993). Action research and quality of care: A mechanism for agreeing basic values as a precursor to change. *Journal of Advanced Nursing, 18,* 305-311.

Peters, T., & Robinson, V. (1984). The origins and status of action research. *Journal of Applied Behavior Science, 20,* 113-124.

Reason, P. (1988). Human inquiry in action: Developments in new paradigm research. London: Sage.

Sheehan, J. (1990). Investigating change in a nursing context. *Journal of Advanced Nursing, 15,* 819-824.

Smith, G. (1986). Resistance to change in geriatric care. *International Journal of Nursing Studies, 23,* 61-70.

Webb, C. (1989). Action research: Philosophy, methods and personal experience. *Journal of Advanced Nursing, 14,* 403-410.

Whyte, F. W. (1991). *Participatory action research.* London: Sage.

17

Poststructuralist Science

An Historical Account of Profound Visibility

LAURA COX DZUREC

Basic elements and the rules by which they are combined—that is the stuff of structuralist science (Dreyfus & Rabinow, 1983). Science is a body of knowledge. On that, both structuralists and poststructuralists might agree. The qualities of that body of knowledge, however, are grist for the mill of contemplation that separates structuralist science from poststructuralist science. In the context of this chapter, structuralist science is considered to be both empiricism and phenomenology.

The ultimate goal of structuralist scientists is to disclose insights into things in the world, to seek truth and meaning. For poststructuralists, science is about something else altogether. Poststructuralists do not acknowledge the existence of grounding laws sought by empiricists or of basic essences or metaphysical truths sought by phenomenologists. Rather, these basic elements, championed by structuralist scientists as the foundation of science, are regarded by poststructuralists as merely a function of what *could* evolve given the political situation at any point in time. For poststructuralists, there is nothing but politics.

A poststructuralist stance is consistent with Shakespeare's notion from *As You Like It* (Craig, 1961): "All the world's a stage, and all the men and women merely players." The aim of poststructuralists is to illustrate the political realities that direct life experiences, to "record the singularity of events outside of any monotonous finality" (Foucault, 1971, p. 138), to overview and recognize that the depth sought by structuralist scientists is no more than "an absolutely superficial secret" (Foucault, 1967, p. 187).

This chapter concerns the rationale and purpose for conducting poststructuralist research. The political issues that poststructuralists are concerned with become the focus of research as the researcher considers people involved with each other in relations of power. What the poststructuralist scientist observes is "subjection, domination, and combat" (Foucault, 1979, p. 26), a play of wills that is the *more factual motivation* for behaviors *said to be emanating* from goodness and altruism.

The Play of Wills:
An Asimov Illustration

Dreyfus and Rabinow (1983) summarized the poststructuralist perspective: The poststructuralist "studies the emergence of a battle which defines and clears a space, . . . subjects emerge on a field of battle and play their roles, there and there alone. The world is not a play *which simply masks a truer reality that exists behind the scenes.* It is as it appears" (p. 109, emphasis added).

In a science fiction novel, Asimov (1985) concisely illustrated the force of the play of wills. His story is summarized as follows:

On a distant-to-earth planet in the future, at least 16 decades after travelers from earth began space exploration, two robots assigned to guard a human's residence talk about the well-being of their human master. The robots—Giskard and Daneel—like all robots, behave in a manner absolutely bound by a basic law of robotics: "A robot may not injure a human being, or through inaction, allow a human being to come to harm" (p. 22).

The laws of robotics, developed by human beings so that robots would not, ultimately, threaten the supremacy of their human masters, are obeyed by all robots. Bound by these laws, Giskard muses, "Intellectually, I think they (the laws of robotics) must be incomplete or insufficient, but when I try to *believe that*, I, too, fail, for I am bound by them. Yet, if I were not bound by them, I am sure I would believe in their insufficiency" (p. 22).

Giskard's dilemma summarizes a notion central to a poststructuralist perspective. At any given time, practices—rules of behavior that support subjection, domination and combat—limit what can be counted as legitimate knowledge. These rules of behavior, in all their inherent political superficiality, absolutely determine what can be known. Such limitation is not, as one might think, the function of primal origins or of unchanging truths. Rather, it is the function of profoundly visible relations of force.

It is the goal of poststructuralists to look at the subjugation inherent in situations involving individuals, who are but pawns of the strategies in operation. Through his comments, Giskard demonstrated how his thinking and acting were absolutely dominated by the play of human will manifested through the laws of robotics. Giskard was bound by human-made laws to protect human beings. His own well-being was subject to the well-being of those he served unquestioningly.

Power/Knowledge

For poststructuralists, knowledge is not synonymous with the factual data considered essential to a discipline. Indeed, according to poststructuralists, factual data DO NOT EXIST. Instead, knowledge is synonymous with layers of clandestine assumptions that shape the interpretation of "facts" and are, more appropriately, intended to maintain established power relations, sustaining fixed social, economic, and political hierarchies.

Recognizing that knowledge is nothing beyond interpretations imposed by power is important to understanding poststructuralism. For poststructuralists, interpreting meanings inherent in raw data to clarify those data is foolish because every situation is inherently meaningless: "There is absolutely nothing primary to interpret because, when all is said and done, underneath it all everything is already interpretation (of the currently-operative plays of will)" (Foucault, 1967, p. 189).

In the Asimov (1985) example, robot Giskard began to question the limiting aspects of the laws of robotics. As a consequence of that consideration, he also began to question what else might exist, what could be, beyond the structure of the laws of robotics that confined his behavior. Giskard's discovery illustrates a second notion important in poststructuralism: As plays of will limit knowledge, they simultaneously encompass productive forces that bring about new knowledge.

Foucault (1967) coined a term—power/knowledge—to address the simultaneous limiting and productive forces of plays of will, and Dzurec (1989) discussed the limiting and productive influences of these plays of will on the development of nursing knowledge. By virtue of its limiting and productive aspects, power/knowledge covertly encourages behavior that is overtly forbidden.

In nursing, for example, the limiting and productive aspects of power/knowledge are illustrated in nurse researchers' increasing willingness to acknowledge multiple paradigms as bases for the conduct of investigation. The process of increasing legitimacy for multiple ways of knowing in nursing evolved as follows.

Historically, legitimate nursing research was couched in the empiricist paradigm. Nonempiricist research approaches such as phenomenology, hermeneutics, grounded theory, and feminism were shunned in serious nursing circles. A network of plays of will (empiricist assumptions promulgated as the only legitimate way to do science) *limited* nursing researchers' ability to know about other kinds of research approaches and effectively held researchers' behaviors and thoughts hostage. Through this network, empiricist researchers maintained their relative power base. Nursing students, practitioners, and researchers were expected to reflect established empirical standards in their work.

However, intimately linked with the limiting forces of power/knowledge were productive forces. In nursing research, the productive forces of power/knowledge were manifested in the sudden proliferation of nonempiricist research. Nurse researchers' interest in historically unacceptable, nonempiricist research methods grew despite, and probably because of, mandated empiricist research in, for example, nursing dissertations, fundable projects, and written reports of nursing investigations. Nurses found that they had good reason to do nonempiricist research and that it was interesting and enjoyable. The notions of intuition and caring, hardly notions consistent with an empiricist viewpoint, became important in clinical work, nursing education, and research. Empiricist claims that nothing but empiricism would do to advance nursing science were met, surprisingly, with retorts that there were other, possibly more appropriate, ways of knowing.

Like nurses, every individual in society is subject to the limiting and productive forces of power/knowledge. However, not all are consciously aware of those forces. Individuals' nescience of these forces is vital to the maintenance of the networks that subjugate individuals. In fact, secrecy is an important influence for the maintenance of networks of power.

Instruments of Discipline

One might ask how power networks are maintained, as over time more and more individuals become aware of them. One set of techniques used to maintain secrecy and preserve the relational networks that limit thinking and behavior is instruments of discipline. Foucault (see Rabinow, 1984) described three instruments of discipline (punishment) used by disciplines (branches of knowledge). These three instruments— examination, normalizing judgment, and hierarchical observation— are employed to maintain existing power relations and to produce "legitimate" knowledge through control and regulation.

The first instrument of discipline, examination, which endorses examinees' depth of knowledge and simultaneously controls the domain of that knowledge, serves a limiting function typical of all three instruments of discipline. One's success on an examination ensures that the individual meets criteria imposed by the extant network. If one fails to succeed on an examination—whether a pencil-and-paper test, a physical inspection, a performance evaluation, or other trial—one is subjected to normalizing judgment, the second instrument of discipline.

Normalizing judgment is comparison of an individual with normative standards for the purpose of maintaining acceptable standards. As one fails to meet those standards, little punishments—for example, bad grades, mandated exercise programs, or more time in the practice lab— are doled out to encourage compliance with acceptable standards. Ultimately, these judgments enhance the vitality with which the extant network of power relations can exert its power over individuals.

The third instrument of discipline is hierarchical observation. Hierarchical observation is constituted by a network that allows individuals at the apex of the extant power structure to view the activities of individuals in all directions. From this panopticon, those with power can further support the power structure and delimit power/knowledge as they see fit. Examples of hierarchical observation include disciplinary research seminars, preparation of papers for disciplinary journals, and disciplinary degree-granting programs. Note the multiple meanings or "multivocity" of the term "disciplinary," simultaneously suggesting wisdom and limitation. Such is the nature of the domain of a poststructuralist.

Instruments of discipline are successful if they maintain the extant power structure. By making examples of individuals who do not conform, those in positions of power limit power/knowledge through the instruments of discipline. However, at the same time that instruments of discipline limit, they suggest to individuals ways in which the extant power structure might be changed. It is through accidental awareness that individuals' developing power/knowledge leads them to question the limitations of the extant power structure. At this juncture, individuals—those who have been subjugated by the operant power structure and those who seek to study that power structure— can come to recognize, instead, the productive potential of their own situation within that power structure.

Asimov's (1985) Giskard, our robotic example, experienced this shift in his understanding of the laws of robotics when confronted with a paradox. To protect one human being, he had to harm many. To obey the absolutely restricting laws of robotics, he had to defy those same laws. The network of relations imposed by the laws left him no choice.

Forced to stand figuratively beyond the restricting laws of robotics, Giskard experienced the productive force inherent in power/knowledge. From a poststructuralist perspective, he devised the Zeroeth law: "Prevention of harm to human beings in groups and to humanity as a whole comes before prevention of harm to any specific individual" (p. 379). Giskard experienced the productive force of power/knowledge.

Similarly, in nursing, researchers who believed patients needed something other than what empiricist methods had to offer also experienced the productive force of power/knowledge. These researchers stood figuratively beyond the restricting assumptions of empiricism to recognize the value of nonempiricist methods to nursing knowledge. As a result of their efforts to broaden the assumptions of legitimacy in nursing, nursing practice, teaching, and research again focused on empirically unmeasurable phenomena such as intuition, caring, suffering, spirituality, and support. Patients reaped the benefits of multiple ways of knowing.

Situating Poststructuralist Science

Poststructuralism is an outgrowth of two philosophies of science: phenomenology and hermeneutics (Dreyfus & Rabinow, 1983). Phenomenologists attempted to make the transcendental turn, bracketing what they knew as they approached things in the world to see those things "as they present themselves in prescientific experience and as they present themselves prior to their scientific interpretation" (Gurwitsch, 1974, p. 17). Hermeneuticists argued for historicality, contending that people cannot use bracketing to divorce themselves from their pasts as they situate themselves in the world in which they live (Ricoeur, 1981).

Both phenomenology and hermeneutics are about meaning situated within a structure. For phenomenologists, the structure is experience. For hermeneuticists, the structure is language. Philosophers in both paradigms champion the context dependence of meaning, despite paradigmatic differences in their approaches to apprehending meaning. The context dependence of meaning valued by both phenomenologists and hermeneuticists is in contrast to the generalizable meaning sought by empiricists, who ultimately would hope to describe phenomena with nomothetic laws. However, the value of meaning for philosophers of all three of these structuralist camps is diametrically opposed to the poststructuralist position on meaning.

Poststructuralist philosophers take issue with meaning altogether, maintaining that everything is meaningless and is a political accident. Dreyfus and Rabinow (1983) summarized the poststructuralist position regarding meaning: The deepest secret that a poststructuralist philosopher has to reveal is that things "have no essence, or that their essence was fabricated in a piecemeal fashion from alien forms" (Foucault, 1971, p. 142). In other words, what appears to be essential about a phenomenon is, more accurately, a function of the play of wills dominating thought about that phenomenon as it evolved over time. To poststructuralists, there are no deep truths, no basic realities. What underlies assumptions are more assumptions. According to poststructuralists, "the universals of our humanism are revealed as the result of the contingent emergence of imposed interpretations" (Dreyfus & Rabinow, 1983, p. 108). Knowledge does not develop because it is available to develop. It develops as a function of power relations, strategic positions held by the players in relationship to each other. Knowledge IS power.

A poststructuralist might have had helpful advice for Giskard, the robot: Struggle not with significance of the laws of robotics but with the will of the humans who imposed the laws of robotics. The content of the laws is inconsequential. The power plays of their authors is all, simultaneously limiting and empowering the individuals subjugated by them. Pay attention to who is making the laws and to whose good those laws serve.

The Historical Account: Doing Poststructuralist Science

Poststructuralist science is constituted by the stories told by individuals in the context of the rules that determine what those stories will entail. Doing poststructuralist science mandates a willingness to let go of essences and to look behind assumptions to other assumptions, never intending to apprehend truth. The poststructuralist scientist will recognize that everything is a political accident that can be viewed in its fullness through examination of the predominance of will.

Poststructuralist science does not disclose the truth or falsehood of information; rather, "it does provide a diagnostic device whereby we can begin to differentiate and locate the functions of different types of discourse" (Dreyfus & Rabinow, 1983, p. 117). Knowledge is NOT subjective or objective. It is, instead, "a central component in the historical transformation of various regimes of power and truth" (Rabinow, 1983, p. 117); it is power. The focus of poststructuralist science is not truth or meaning because there IS NO TRUTH OR MEANING. Recognizing the absence of meaning as an aspect of any phenomenon, the poststructuralist focuses on discourse: dialogue between people in the network of power relations. The goal is to evaluate the claim of that discourse to describe reality.

A first step in using poststructuralist methods is to look beyond the assumptions that ground any given science or that ground the scientist personally. Questioning assumptions is a particularly vital step in the poststructuralist process. Taking this step requires that one recognize that science is, indeed, grounded in assumptions and then stand figuratively beyond those assumptions to recognize their impact on the practice of science. Scientists practicing without recognizing that science is grounded in assumptions, a naive perspective, are practicing "scientism." Paradoxically, those practicing scientism tend to believe that their science is SCIENCE and everything else a sham. For individuals operating from scientism, the network of power relations is most successful at maintaining secrecy and limiting knowledge.

A second step in the conduct of poststructuralist science is to recognize that grounding interpretation is deeper-level interpretation. The poststructuralist constantly questions assumptions that supposedly "found" ideas, considering what discourse allowed those ideas to flourish as they evolved in time. Truth is not a function of the quality of one's approach to science or of metaphysics but of discourse and of power.

The third step in poststructuralist analysis is to acknowledge that there is nothing to know, in the sense that one understands a body of knowledge and its attendant theoretical accoutrements. There is only discourse that creates knowledge. The goal of poststructuralist science is to describe phenomena as they appear—not in the sense that a phenomenologist or hermeneuticist would attempt this description but in a manner that describes the play of forces operating at any point in time.

A fourth step in the method is to acknowledge that the individual is forever subjugated by the power relations inherent in the network of relations. The individual subject is the absolute limit of power, and the body is the site at which the power of the network of relations is demonstrated. Instruments of discipline are used on individuals to show the larger mass of subjects the power position of the network of relations. This show of power helps to maintain the status quo.

Yet the poststructuralist recognizes, in using the steps of the method, that power/knowledge both limits and enables knowledge development. Poststructuralist analysis is directed toward situating a theory of discourse (archaeology) within a theory of power (genealogy).

Archaeology and Genealogy

In his early writings, Foucault focused on archaeology, that is, on examination of the structure of interaction in the tradition of hermeneuticists. After 1968, Foucault's focus shifted to genealogy, the theory of power. Foucault's early interest in archaeology was an outgrowth of his value for hermeneutics. As his work in poststructuralist analysis continued, Foucault concentrated less and less on the analysis of discourse and become more concerned with the rules directing that discourse (Dreyfus & Rabinow, 1983).

Thus, as it has evolved, poststructuralist analysis focuses on the genealogy of objectifying trends in a culture: the power relations that maintain the hierarchical social structure. To study these trends, one examines subjectifying practices, that is, practices that point a powerful, controlling finger at individuals who fail to conform to norms of the network of power relations. Because individuals are the carriers of the norms and rules of the operant power network, understanding the political forces by which those rules and norms are conveyed to individuals is the crux of poststructuralist science. Studying the rules directing the discourse of the power network shows the nature of truth to be nothing more than political power.

Ricoeur (1982) argued that hermeneutics is the science of science by virtue of its goal of understanding meaning. Poststructuralist philosophers would argue that poststructuralism is broader yet, incorporating norms, rules, and systems that limit power/knowledge. The poststructuralists, of course, deny the inherent meaning that hermeneuticists seek to unearth. Instead, a poststructuralist "seeks to establish a set of flexible relationships, and merge them into a single apparatus in order to isolate a specific historical problem. This apparatus brings together power and knowledge into a specific grid of analysis" (Dreyfus & Rabinow, 1983, p. 121).

Data for a poststructuralist analysis include language, discursive meaning within a political context and subjectivity. The poststructuralist is constantly aware of the subjugation of the individual by the operative relations of power. The research strategy involves studying phenomena as they are enmeshed in cultural practices through a method that shows how extant truth is merely a component of modern power (Dreyfus & Rabinow, 1983, p. 120).

Relationship to Practice

Clearly, the fundamental theme in poststructuralism is the intimate connection between the production of knowledge and the exercise of power. Control and delimitation regulate discourse and hence knowledge. The nurse researcher using poststructuralist analysis will abandon knowledge claims based in structuralist science and question instead how a phenomenon evolved within a political context. At issue is not truth and meaning, which for poststructuralists do not exist, but power relations. Poststructuralist analysis will not shed light on the content of nursing's knowledge domain because, according to poststructuralists, there is no knowledge domain. Instead, poststructuralist research will offer elucidation of the layers of assumptions that are the basis of "knowledge" in a given discipline.

Such a stance is important to nursing, itself a youthful discipline whose practitioners are predominantly female. Practicing nurses often find that their patients do not fit with standards maintained by extant knowledge claims. Poststructuralists would charge those nurses with examination of the theories and postulates that nursing scientists hold dear to identify whether they are adequate in their description of "reality."

Poststructuralist analysis of nursing's phenomena of concern poses critical questions for evaluation. Are the phenomena of interest to nurses what they seem to be? Muller and Dzurec (1993) asked this question, asserting that what has been held to constitute maternal-fetal attachment and mental illness in recent decades might be suspect. The popular terms that characterized these nursing phenomena were more a vehicle for the advancement of narrow views than a comprehensive portrayal of what, indeed, constituted the phenomena.

What will the network of power relations allow with regard to the development of nursing knowledge? These are important issues that mandate a comprehensive description of the phenomena of concern to nursing.

Foucault argued that he was not a poststructuralist (Dreyfus & Rabinow, 1983, pp. vi-vii). He recognized that there were paradoxes inherent in poststructuralism. Two particularly problematic paradoxes are the poststructuralists' reliance on theory and on hermeneutics. Specifically, to maintain that one is atheoretical automatically situates one within a theory (a theory of atheory); to interpret discourse automatically situates one within a hermeneutic stance. However, poststructuralism offers nurse researchers an opportunity to evaluate claims of truth from a perspective that is beyond the limitations of traditional science, to recognize the power of knowledge and the knowledge of power.

Foucault and other poststructuralists are not unaware of the problems inherent in a poststructuralist perspective. They recognize that they, like all of us, are simultaneously produced and subjugated by the very power relations under study. Yet to take a poststructuralist stance is to interpret phenomena in their fullness, to create a historical account of profound visibility.

Dickson (1990) used a poststructuralist stance to evaluate knowledge of menopause. Through her analysis, Dickson challenged dominant beliefs about "truths" surrounding menopause, making the genealogy of menopause apparent. Dzurec (1994) asked questions about the power experiences of people with schizophrenia. The following chapter demonstrates the process of that inquiry, presenting a poststructuralist analysis of the assumptions that have grounded scientists in their quest to uncover causes for severe mental disability.

References

Asimov, I. (1985). *Robots and empire.* New York: Doubleday.

Craig, H. (1961). *The complete works of Shakespeare.* Chicago: Scott, Foresman.

Dickson, G. L. (1990). A feminist poststructuralist analysis of the knowledge of menopause. *Advances in Nursing Science, 12*(3), 15-31.

Dreyfus, H. L., & Rabinow, P. (1983). *Michel Foucault: Beyond structuralism and hermeneutics.* Chicago: University of Chicago Press.

Dzurec, L. C. (1989). The necessity and evolution of multiple paradigms for nursing research: A poststructuralist perspective. *Advances in Nursing Science, 11*(4), 69-79.

Dzurec, L. C. (1994). Schizophrenic clients' experiences of power: A hermeneutic analysis. *Image: The Journal of Nursing Scholarship, 26,* 157-161.

Foucault, M. (1967). Nietzsche, Freud and Marx. In Colloque Philosophique International de Royaumont (Ed.), *Nietzsche* (pp. 183-192). Paris: Editions de Minuit.

Foucault, M. (1971). Nietzsche, genealogy, and history. In D. F. Bouchard (Ed.), *Michel Foucault: Language, counter-memory, practice. Selected essays and interviews* (S. Simon, Trans.; pp. 139-164). New York: Cornell University Press.

Foucault, M. (1979). *Discipline and punish: The birth of the prison* (A. Sheridan, Trans.). New York: Random House.

Gurwitsch, A. (1974). *Phenomenology and the theory of science.* Evanston, IL: Northwestern University Press.

Muller, M. E., & Dzurec, L. C. (1993). The power of THE NAME. *Advances in Nursing Science, 15*(3), 15-22.

Rabinow, P. (1984). *The Foucault reader.* New York: Pantheon.

Ricoeur, P. (1981). *Hermeneutics and the human sciences* (J. B. Thompson, Trans.). Cambridge: Cambridge University Press.

18

Severe Mental Disability?
Or a Play of Wills?

LAURA COX DZUREC

To be considered severely and chronically mentally ill has never been a position of privilege. In differing social and temporal contexts, physical brutality, exclusion, neglect, punishment, and confinement have been prescribed as "treatment" for severely mentally ill people. Varying and sometimes overlapping perspectives have dictated both social consideration and clinical management of the mentally ill across time and across cultures (Haber, Leach McMahon, Price-Hoskins, & Sideleau, 1992; Wilson & Kneisl, 1988).

Efforts to understand and contend with mental illness proceed through such endeavors as education of health care providers, advancements in technology, and the development of new psychoactive medications. Yet despite the directed efforts of health care professionals from every realm—physicians, nurses, counselors, social workers, biomedical engineers, psychologists—mental illness has defied definition

245

and treatment. People with mental disability have benefited litle in terms of cure (Bachrach, 1980; Lidz, 1990).

Poststructuralism offers avenues for study of the knowledge claims surrounding mental disability, its causes, and its ramifications. From this perspective, severe mental disability can be understood in terms of its value-laden assumptions and circumstances. It is these assumptions and circumstances—and not the characteristics of mental disability itself—that absolutely limit knowledge regarding severe mental disability. The systematic and simultaneous study of the "special population" of mentally ill clients, treatment resources, public policy, and political and social realities constitute the core of poststructuralist study of severe mental disability.

The aim of this chapter is to examine the assumptions that circumscribe severe mental disability and to show them as a source of treatment failures. From a poststructuralist perspective, the nature of severe mental disability can be elucidated through recognition of the value-laden assumptions that impel it.

Historical Overview of Severe Disability Management

Mental illness and its treatment have a long history in the United States, primarily involving institutional care for the mentally ill. As a consequence of the emotional traumas suffered by soldiers in World War II, ideas regarding appropriate treatment of mental illness changed.

In the early 1960s, the President's Commission on Mental Illness and Mental Health (Joint Commission on Mental Illness and Health, 1961) was established to support study of the community mental health movement. This movement was fueled by a more than 100-year history of asylum treatment failures (Elpers, 1987; Smoyak, 1991) and a political emphasis on individuals' rights that grew from strong civil libertarian pressure during an era of sociopolitical reform (Bachrach, 1976). Additionally, the early 1950s marked the discovery of psychotropic drugs that rendered previously unmanageable patients docile (French, 1987), hence contributing to the view that mental illness was a neurophysiological phenomenon.

Events of World War II, clinical research, and the political climate conjointly blended to provide legislators and deinstitutionalization proponents with evidence that state mental institution policies and practices were not optimal for treating mental illness (Elpers, 1987; Osborne & Thomas, 1991; Smoyak, 1991). Sanctioned by mental health professionals who championed the view that severe mental disability was indeed a biomedical problem and by legislation such as the National Mental Health Act of 1946, the Mental Health Study Act of 1955, and the Mental Retardation Facilities and Community Mental Health Centers Construction Act of 1963, the community mental health movement and the concept of deinstitutionalization continued to flourish over time. Mounting criticism regarding the involuntary nature of psychiatric hospitalization fostered development of the notion of mental health treatment in the least restrictive environment (French, 1987; Luskin, 1983; Wilson, 1987). However, effective community treatment, including prevention, early intervention, and rehabilitation, was not accessible (Pepper, 1987; Wilson, 1987). Resources and commitment promised at the national level during the 1960s were not delivered (James, 1987). Families of mentally ill individuals often were overburdened and felt defeated in their efforts to provide care in an environment that offered limited professional support and inadequate legal, social, and clinical controls on mentally ill patients (Elpers, 1987). Legislation couched in least restrictive environment rhetoric allowed discharged patients to refuse treatment of any kind unless they posed imminent threat to themselves or others (French, 1989; Wilson, 1987).

A network of community-based resources developed in response to federal mandates for treatment of severely mentally ill individuals in environments of least restriction. However, these resourses were inadequate: More and more unexpected physiological and behavioral problems developed in clients (Bachrach, 1992; Pepper, 1987), families became increasingly unsure of their roles and responsibilities for care and found unclear support for their efforts (Bassuk & Buckner, 1992), and communities, sheltered from the mentally ill for more than 100 years by institutional walls, were not ready to live among the mentally ill (Hanson & Rapp, 1992). As the number of state mental hospital beds decreased, the number of correctional facility beds grew (French, 1989). Some states considered legislation that would mandate repeated one-year commitments for persons whose initial violent crime was caused or aggravated by a mental illness (Elpers, 1987).

Lack of financial support from the federal government and state mandates for balanced state budgets fueled an ongoing imbalance between client, family, and community needs and available resources. Individual states began taking over mental health care as early as 1962 as a result of the Mental Health Study Act of 1955. Subsequent legislation such as the Drug Export Amendments Act of 1982 continued this trend as the federal economy turned downward. Scarce resources served as yet another source of problems in the implementation of deinstitutionalization (James, 1987; Ross, Mazade, & Cohen, 1992).

Despite legislation mandating them, treatment options for the severely mentally disabled decreased over the course of time. Deinstitutionalization, community treatment, neurophysiological interventions, and legislation—interventions that made abundant theoretical sense—did not solve the problems of severely mentally disabled people. As Zealberg (1988) asserted, the people most in need of cutting-edge psychiatry—those with severe mental disability—were (and are) the people least likely to receive it. For example, a "breakthrough" such as clozapine, a recently developed antipsychotic, was not available to people with severe mental disability who had few advocates and fewer functional organized systems of care (McFarland, 1992).

From a poststructuralist perspective, severe mental disability provides an exemplary stage for the play of wills. The viscissitudes of severe mental disability are no more than a function of "the contingent emergence of imposed interpretations" (Dreyfus & Rabinow, 1983, p. 108). For poststructuralists, the problems couching severe mental disability can be understood NOT in terms of inadequate understanding of the phenomenon of severe mental disability but in terms of the influence of circumscribing presuppositions. Two assumptions—a conceptualization of severe mental disability as neuropathophysiological in nature and the societal values that reinforce such a conceptualization—are the focus of this analysis.

Legitimate Knowledge Regarding Severe Mental Disability: Neuropathophysiology

The notion that severe mental disability is physiologic in nature has been a major factor influencing the direction of thinking about and treatment for severe mental disability. The relations between mind and brain have been the subject of intensive debate encompassing volumes of philosophical literature. The mind-brain debate emanated from theological beginnings and continued over the centuries, with multiple themes emerging as scientists attempted to understand the connection between the mind and brain (Churchland, 1986; Harrington, 1987). Certainly, the debate continues in philosphical circles (Blakemore & Greenfield, 1987; Kenny, 1992). The current focus in the clinical treatment of severe mental disability is on the brain, a perspective fueled by legislative mandates and patterns of funding that support neurophysiological research.

The neurophysiological research is compelling. Zealberg (1988), for example, identified components of "cutting edge" psychiatry as "physiology of the locus coeruleus, of G proteins as they relate to receptors, and of how interleukins affect cortisol production" (p. 1544). The dopamine hypothesis has been advanced as an explanation for schizophrenia (Meltzer, 1987; Thompson, 1990). Viruses and autoimmunity have been implicated in severe mental disability as well.

Yet years of research have determined nothing certain. For example, although research has shown that there are, indeed, lesions in the brains of people with severe mental disability, similar research has shown that those lesions are present in the brains of people *without* severe mental disability (Mesulam, 1990). Such discrepancy suggests, as Lidz (1990) noted, that the optimism expressed by mental health professionals regarding the potential discovery of a physiological etiology for mental illness is premature, that some other (albeit inadmissible) problem is operative for people with severe mental disability. Furthermore, clinical observation demonstrates that despite a rapidly expanding body of neurophysiological knowledge and accompanying protracted biomedical interventions, the severely mentally disabled continue to have the same problems they have had historically. Such discrepancy also suggests the narrow limits imposed by neurophysiologic power/ knowledge. As Lidz (1990) noted, although these breakthroughs have told us much about neurophysiology, they have told us virtually nothing about severe mental disability.

The instruments of discipline—examination, normalizing judgments, and hierarchical observation—have served a limiting function in the evolution of power/knowledge regarding severe mental disability, facilitating the growth of physiologically based arguments for severe mental disability. There is little serious regard for nonphysiological explanations of severe mental disability; there is little reason to afford other explanations serious regard in the absence of funding, support, and collegiality and in the presence of potential professional scorn. Because of funding patterns, health professionals' education regarding severe mental disability has been physiological in nature. *Examination* (paper-and-pencil tests, practice in completing histories and physicals) has ensured that health professionals understand the neurophysiologic basis of mental disability. *Normalizing judgment* (passing coursework in psychiatry, obtaining funding for research) has maintained the physiologically based line of thought regarding severe mental disability. *Hierarchical observation* (presenting or publishing findings, serving as a teacher in severe mental disability) has guaranteed that only physiology would convey as new students learned about severe mental disability.

Yet making mental illness a problem with a pathophysiological cause has been attributed with certain anticipated advantages ("What Are Your Feelings?," 1988). These advantages are among the productive outcomes of the power/knowledge of severe mental disability. According to some, biomedicalization of mental illness alters societal acceptance of the problem, limiting associated stigma for clients. Concurrently, biomedicalization provides mental health professionals with tools that they could use to enhance the well-being of affected clients. Remarkable reversals in behavior of affected patients are said to occur (and have occurred spasmodically) following biomedical interventions.

Fox and Chamberlain (1988) and McBride (1990) noted that the biomedicalization of mental illness provides opportunities for interdisciplinary attempts to cure mental illness. By virtue of the number and diversity of their contributors, interdisciplinary rather than unidisciplinary endeavors would seem to offer relatively more potential rewards.

The medical literature is replete with arguments for and research about new findings that support the argument that mental illness has a physiological etiology. Meltzer (1987) cited an "explosion of information" (p. v) regarding developments in psychopharmacology—a consequence of a huge increase in neuroscientists and a not-so-huge-but-notable increase in clinical investigators—as the rationale for a major revision of his extensive and comprehensive psychopharmacology text. Drug companies have increased the sizes of their research staffs ("New Drugs," 1988), and development of new drugs is ongoing.

However, touted advantages notwithstanding, maintaining severe mental disability as a neurophysiological problem has ensured the well-being of the nondisabled, keeping them comfortably apart from the mentally ill. In concert with the instruments of discipline, a deeply entrenched system of values and a well-established economic system have also served to maintain the structure of severe mental disability power/knowledge and sustain inherent problems.

Value-Laden Assumptions: Economics, Semantics, and Attitudes

Failures in the treatment of people with severe mental disability can be traced, in measurable part, to unspoken values that pervade American life and constitute profoundly visible yet hidden assumptions that drive thinking and action concerning severe mental disability. An assumption of scarcity motivates mental health care (and the entire health care system) (Illich, 1982). Concern over scarcity of resources has spawned a value system favoring work over welfare, upward over downward mobility, high over low status, independence over dependence, individualism over collectivity, moralism over immorality, and ascription over blamelessness (Tropman, 1989). Scarce resources are allocated to those worthy of them, to those whose beliefs and actions correspond with accepted values.

Severely mentally disabled individuals, according to the circumscribing assumptions, are physiologically incapable of worth. They have difficulty holding jobs. They are, at best, laterally mobile, notably poor in asserting their individuality, dependent, and potentially immoral. However, the same physiology that renders them relatively valueless also renders them blameless—they cannot be held responsible for their physiology. This paradox spawned the protracted clinical, social, and legislative efforts characterizing the history of severe mental disability and its treatment (a productive outcome of power/ knowledge).

Although efforts have indeed resulted in the removal of physical barriers (walls) and social barriers (access) and resulted even in the development (albeit erratic and fragmented) of formalized, institutionalized community resources, they have not and will not change the attitude component of deinstitutionalization. Unchecked, this attitude has simultaneously directed a backlash of processes designed specifically (if with societal naïveté) to reconstruct personal barriers to mentally ill individuals, to effectively segregate them, to keep them out of sight and out of mind (Bassuk & Buckner, 1992).

Both sides of the paradox are played out: The severely mentally disabled are blameless for their physiology and warrant resources; however, despite their blamelessness, the severely mentally disabled are unworthy of scarce and shrinking resources. One can choose to defend either side by virtue of the complex semantics inherent in power/ knowledge regarding severe mental disability. Not surprising, semantic paradoxes surface over and over in regard to severe mental disability as the paradoxical value system is played out.

For example, Bachrach (1976) introduced clinicians to the semantics of deinstitutionalization, noting that the term "institution" refers not only to *physical place* but also to *sets of social patterns*. Place and social pattern are not mutually exclusive domains of institutionalization; rather, they are hierarchical outcomes of a mitigating variable—attitude.

An attitude is a fixed belief. People living together in social groups share attitudes, developing consensual social patterns, such as values, that extend from those attitudes. Physical structures reflecting attitudes and social patterns are created to embody and formalize attitudes. Attitudes subsequently become fixed to those physical places, and change in attitudes, once they are formalized in physical structures, comes slowly, more or less as a function of splinter groups who introduce new attitudes to challenge those that are established.

Such was the pattern resulting in the deinstitutionalization and community treatment stance that evolved for people with severe mental disabilities. Concerned individuals acting on the attitude that people with severe mental disabilities are blameless poured extensive, well-intentioned effort into alternative therapies, but the process— while removing barriers and walls—did not deter social institutionalization. For example, in many communities, the threat of "group home" is met with anger, resistance, and political action; patrons in restaurants complain if mentally ill people disturb their dinners; town managers are contacted to force mentally ill people living in the streets to refrain from bothering citizens who reside nearby.

Yet another paradox confronts those who would banish the severely mentally disabled. With the intent of protecting the mentally ill, legislation has made it difficult for them to get needed inpatient treatment.

Involuntary hospitalization is a route of last resort in an economically limited environment in which providers, consumers, and family members favor least restrictive treatment alternatives. However, because community resources have been slowly developed and remain generally underdeveloped, there are no treatment options for many severely disabled people.

In short, paradoxical, value-laden assumptions that impel power/ knowledge have resulted in an impasse for people with severe mental disability and for the nondisabled as well. The severely mentally disabled have never truly moved beyond the institution, a structure that, even in the absence of material presence, formalizes values and couches power/knowledge regarding severe mental disability.

Institutions

Institutions, useful in maintaining mentally ill persons' positions of relative worthlessness and, in so doing, maintaining the relative worth of people who are not mentally ill, fix attitudes. They are the formal mechanism by which scarce resources are allocated. Institutions historically have served to formalize the efficient and fixed value system of a society that must allocate scarce resources, including economic resources, appropriately. They support the social and physical segregation of people who only scarcely deserve already scarce resources. They streamline the complex process of deciding who shall have and who shall not. Institutions, in short, serve an important, controlling, economic function. The institution symbolizes the paradoxical values that drive thinking about severe mental disability.

"Every modern institution, from school to family and from union to courtroom, incorporates . . . [the] . . . assumption of scarcity" (Illich, 1982, p. 11). For example, education is the institution by which individuals learn that qualifications and competence are scarce goods for which all must compete. Similarly, mental health treatment (institutionalization) is the institution by which individuals learn that sanity and normal behavior are scarce goods for which all must compete. Institutions maintain social structure; they support "invidious individualism" (Illich, 1982, p. 12), engendering economic competition in a society in which some must invariably serve as the have-not counterpart to those who have.

Mental institutions, once considered optimal in the humane treatment of the mentally ill, fell victim to the lessons of history and experience. Attitudes and social patterns changed regarding hospital treatment of the mentally ill, and a movement toward deinstitutionalization began. However, by virtue of the play of wills operative around assumptions, deinstitutionalization, community treatment, and destigmatization could not be realized. Institutions and their accompanying stigma are part and parcel of the values and economics of American life; the severely mentally disabled, as part of the society, are necessarily constrained by institutions.

Within the shrouded context of value complexity and economic scarcity, there can only be institutions, even if they are without walls. The severely mentally disabled have themselves become an institution, structuring and perpetuating the extant values and economic system characterizing our society.

Recommendations

As they forced deinstitutionalization on an unwilling public, clinical, social, and legislative efforts have resulted in the institutionalization of the mentally ill in places without walls. While pending and ongoing mandates decreed the individualized treatment of people with mental illness, economic scarcity demanded physical and social segregation on the basis of relative worth. The assumptions circumscribing severe mental disability allowed the removal of physical and social barriers and simultaneously motivated the erection of personal barriers.

Although legislation, clinical breakthroughs, and social change were intended to aid people with severe mental disability, their effect was minimal and paradoxical. Efforts to confront and eliminate severe mental disability have been, more accurately (if naively), efforts in service of the assumptions grounding severe mental disability. A play of wills—domination, combat, and subjugation—constitutes the superficial grounds on which "severe mental disability," like all phenomena, rests.

To recognize the limitations imposed by our assumptions is the goal of a poststructuralist scientist. To do the best we can for the person with "severe mental disability," cognizant of the limitations imposed by our assumptions, is the goal of a poststructuralist scientist nurse.

Until the assumptions driving severe mental disability, its conceptualization, and its treatment are clarified and made apparent, more paradoxical and untoward effects of well-intentioned efforts on behalf of the severely mentally disabled will ensue. Programs will be cut and money will be reallocated to more deserving individuals and programs. Indeed, deinstitutionalization itself has not been spared the ravages of scarcity. For example, in light of scarce federal and state resources, scaling back of services (Ross et al., 1992), better organized methods of planning and delivery of mental health care (Hudson, Salloway, & Vissing, 1992), and combinations of both (Sederer, 1992; Surles, Blanch, & Shepardson, 1992) have been proposed. In view of scarcity, some authors have called for mental health professionals' renewed commitment and advocacy in the face of shortage (Duldt, 1991; Gordon, 1990; Hagerty, Lynch-Sauer, Patusky, Bouwsema, & Collier, 1992; James, 1987), whereas still others have called for a proactive rather than a reactive statewide stance in response to legislative mandates (Ross et al., 1992).

However, renewed advocacy is an inadequate solution to the problems of severe mental disability. Affecting the course and outcomes of caring for people with severe mental disability *does* demand efforts such as those that have been undertaken to enhance mentally ill individuals' access to the same rights, responsibilities, and privileges that all other people have. However, to be effective, those efforts must necessarily address the assumptions circumscribing treatment of the mentally ill.

For example, if characteristics of the mentally ill are the subject of legislation (as is currently the case), characteristics of other members of society also should be legislated; alternatively, no one's characteristics might be legislated. Some mental health professionals are speaking out about the negative aspects of the biomedicalization of severe mental disability (Lidz, 1990; Mesulam, 1990; "What Are Your Feelings?," 1988; Zealberg, 1988), suggesting new knowledge that might be incorporated into the domain of severe mental disability. Such effort is laudable and certainly will contribute to appropriate legislation and clinical efforts. No effort will be successful, however, that does not recognize that biomedicalization itself is an institution.

For poststructuralists, there is no knowledge domain; there are no facts; there is no truth. There is only power: relative positions within a society, plays of will acted out in complete superficiality. To search for a cause—biomedical or otherwise—for severe mental disability is a pursuit that is, at best, trivial. Instead, focusing on hidden assumptions is the key to power/knowledge. The interplay of assumptions—manifest as institutions—drives severe mental disability and yields a scenario that, decontextualized, is paradoxical. Care for people with severe mental disability will be enhanced only when mental health professionals take stock of societal values, the attendant interplay of semantics, attitudes, and economics, and a well-reinforced view of severe mental disability as neurophysiological and use that awareness to extend the limits of power/knowledge.

Affecting the course and outcomes of deinstitutionalization does demand social policies such as those that have been enacted to enhance mentally ill individuals' access to the same rights, responsibilities, and privileges that all other people have. However, legislation as it is written addresses only OUTCOMES and FINANCIAL INCENTIVES (competition) for achieving those outcomes. To be effective, social policies must also address the PROCESS of deinstitutionalization. Not only should characteristics of the mentally ill be the subject of legislation (as is currently the case) but also the characteristics of other members of society should be the subject of legislation. Deinstitutionalization cannot be successful in a society in which individuals are not at least cognizant of the needs of all other members of that society (and one might question whether it can be successful at all in a society based on competition and scarcity). From this perspective, the following recommendations are proposed.

First, all individuals will need to feel secure about themselves and their own abilities before deinstitutionalization can be successful. (Is such a scenario possible in a society where one is always readily replaced by someone younger, better educated, and more "cutting edge"?) One way to implement personal efficacy is to mandate that people learn to parent successfully. Research to date suggests that successful parenting involves listening to children, communicating with them, offering them opportunities for open discussion about issues, and teaching them to deal with feelings—a list more comprehensive than could feasibly be presented in the context of this chapter. In any case, it is possible to teach and to learn effective parenting, and to fund the development of additional knowledge about parenting, and this is an important first step to changing the mental health system (assuming that the institutions of parenting do not interfere).

Second, the education of mental health professionals requires more breadth. Particularly, the challenge directed toward an empiricist view, the tenets of which are consistent with competitive capitalistic values, should be continued. Caring can be reintroduced in curricula, as it has been in certain curricula (Duldt, 1991; Gordon, 1990; Hagerty et al., 1992). Ways of knowing that permit knowledge grounded in discovery rather than in verification, in idiosyncrasy rather than in modal tendencies, and in understanding rather than in explanation should supplement knowledge of cause and effect. Such breadth of knowledge enhances recognition of assumptions.

Third, increased exposure of the general public to the mentally ill will desensitize them and prepare them to deal with relevant issues and problems. A media blitz (some of which is already in process) would make the complexities of mental illness common knowledge and challenge existing assumptions. Concomitantly, mental health professionals might consider the paradox of shrouding mental illness in secrecy in the name of maintaining confidentiality.

Fourth, mentally ill people need increased access to health care. Prevention might be enhanced by early detection of physical and emotional problems that are held to result in mental illness. Pending legislation of a national program of health insurance can be organized to assist the mentally ill in their efforts to get treatment. To do less is ludicrous in a context in which physiology is viewed as the sine qua non of severe mental disability.

Fifth, mental health professionals should actively consider the foregoing discussion, for this IS the context of severe mental disability. To free the mentally ill from the physical barriers of institutions and from the social barriers of limited access in the semantic and economic context characterizing mental health care is to necessarily subject them to the personal barriers of attitude. Social policy and clinical efforts must be directed toward anticipating reinstitutionalization at this personal level. Institutionalization will not go away. We cannot legislate it out of existence.

As Krauthammer (1988) noted, "To expect the saintliness of the ordinary citizen is bad social policy. Further, to expose him hourly to a wretchedness far *beyond his power to remedy* is to make moral insensitivity a requirement of daily living" (p. 24, emphasis added). In light of the context of severe mental disability, asking health professionals, family members, or lay people simply to treat the severely mentally disabled humanistically and uniquely is morally insensitive. Treatment mechanisms operative in a complex economy such as that of the United

States mandate normative, not individualized, standards for care. Even now, terminology is shifting from "least restrictive environment" to "most therapeutic environment" as practitioners gear up to respond to the ongoing problems of deinstitutionalization.

Like all social institutions, severe mental disability and its accoutrements are subject to interpretation and implementation for the masses. Until the masses change their way of thinking, the severely mentally disabled will necessarily remain victims of semantic and economic vicissitudes of values.

References

Bachrach, L. L. (1976). *Deinstitutionalization: An analytical review and sociological perspective*. Rockville, MD: U.S. Department of Health Education, and Welfare; Public Health Service; Alcohol, Drug Abuse, and Mental Health Administration.

Bachrach, L. L. (1980). Is the least restrictive environment always the best? Sociological and semantic implications. *Hospital and Community Psychiatry, 31*, 91-103.

Bachrach, L. L. (1992). "The chronic patient": In search of a title. *Hospital and Community Psychiatry, 43*, 867-871.

Bassuk, E. L., & Buckner, J. C. (1992). Out of mind—Out of sight. *American Journal of Orthopsychiatry, 62*, 330-331.

Blakemore, C., & Greenfield, S. (Eds.). (1987). *Mindwaves*. Cambridge, MA: Blackwell.

Churchland, P. (1986). *Neurophilosophy*. Cambridge: MIT Press.

Duldt, B. (1991). "I-Thou" in nursing: Research supporting Duldt's theory. *Perspectives in Psychiatric Care, 27*, 5-12.

Dreyfus, H. L., & Rabinow, P. (1983). *Michel Foucault: Beyond structuralism and hermeneutics*. Chicago: University of Chicago Press.

Elpers, J. R. (1987). Are we legislating reinstitutaionlization? *American Journal of Orthopsychiatry, 57*, 441-446.

Fox, J. C., & Chamberlain, J. (1988). Preparing nurses to work with the chronically mentally ill. *Community Mental Health Journal, 24*(4), 296-309.

French, L. (1987). Victimization of the mentally ill: An unintended consequence of deinstitutionalization. *Social Work, 32*, 502-505.

French, L. (1989). Deinstitutionalization or victimization? A reply to Segal. *Social Work, 34*, 471-472.

Gordon, J. S. (1990). Holistic medicine and mental health practice: Toward a new syntheses. *American Journal of Orthopsychiatry, 60*, 357-369.

Haber, J., Leach McMahon, A., Price-Hoskins, P., & Sideleau, B. F. (1992). *Comprehensive psychiatric nursing* (4th ed.). St. Louis: Mosby.

Hagerty, B. M. K., Lynch-Sauer, J., Patusky, K. L., Bouwsema, M., & Collier, P. (1992). Sense of belonging: A vital mental health concept. *Archives of Psychiatric Nursing, 6*, 172-177.

Hanson, J. C., & Rapp, C. A. (1992). Families' perceptions of community mental health programs for their relatives with severe mental illness. *Community Mental Health Journal, 28,* 181-198.

Harrington, A. (1987). *Medicine, mind and the double brain.* Princeton, NJ: Princeton University Press.

Hudson, C. B., Salloway, J. C., & Vissing, Y. M. (1992). The impact of state administrative practices on community mental health. *Administration and Policy in Mental Health, 19,* 417-436.

Illich, I. (1982). *Gender.* Berkeley, CA: Heyday.

James, J. F. (1987). Does the community mental health movement have the momentum needed to survive? *American Journal of Orthopsychiatry, 57,* 447-451.

Joint Commission on Mental Illness and Health. (1961). *Action for mental health.* New York: Basic Books.

Kenny, A. (1992). *Metaphysics of mind.* Oxford: Oxford University Press.

Krauthammer, C. (1988). How to save the homeless mentally ill. *New Republic, 198*(6), 22-25.

Lidz, T. (1990, March 16). Optimism in treatment of schizophrenia still premature, says expert. *Psychiatric News,* p. 8.

Luskin, R. D. (1983). *Compulsory outpatient treatment for the mentally ill.* Report to the American Psychiatric Association Task Force on Involuntary Outpatient Treatment, Washington, DC.

McBride, A. B. (1990). Psychiatric nursing in the 1990s. *Archives of Psychiatric Nursing, 4*(1), 21-28.

McFarland, B. H. (1992). Discontinuing clozapine: An example of explicit health care rationing. *Administration and Policy in Mental Health, 19,* 399-416.

Meltzer, H. Y. (Ed.). (1987). *Psychopharmacology: The third generation of progress.* New York: Raven Press.

Mesulam, M. M. (1990). Schizophrenia and the brain. *New England Journal of Medicine, 320,* 842-844.

New drugs. (1988, February-March). *NAMI News, 9*(1), 5.

Osborne, O. H., & Thomas, M. D. (1991). On public sector psychosocial nursing: A conceptual framework. *Journal of Psychosocial Nursing, 29*(8), 13-18.

Pepper, B. (1987). A public policy for the long-term mentally ill: A positive alternative to reinstitutionalization. *American Journal of Orthopsychiatry, 57,* 452-457.

Ross, E. C., Mazade, N. A., & Cohen, M. D. (1992). Current tensions in financing public mental health services. *Administration and Policy in Mental Health, 19*(6), 459-465.

Sederer, L. I. (1992). Judicial and legislative responses to cost containment. *American Journal of Psychiatry, 149,* 1157-1161.

Smoyak, S. (1991). Psychosocial nursing in public versus private sectors: An introduction. *Journal of Psychosocial Nursing, 29*(8), 6-12.

Surles, R. C., Blanch, A. K., & Shepardson, J. (1992). Integrating mental health policy, financing, and program development: The New York State experience. *Administration and Policy in Mental Health, 19,* 269-277.

Thompson, L. W. (1990). The dopamine hypothesis of schizophrenia. *Perspectives in Psychiatric Care, 26*(3), 18-23.

Tropman, J. (1989). *American values and social welfare: Cultural contradictions in the welfare state*. Englewood Cliffs, NJ: Prentice Hall.

What are your feelings about the trend toward the biomedicalization of psychiatry? (1988). *Journal of Psychosocial Nursing and Mental Health Services, 26*(1), 40-41.

Wilson, R. D. (1987). *Involuntary civil commitment of the mentally ill in the post-reform era*. Springfield, IL: Charles C Thomas.

Wilson, H. S., & Kneisl, C. R. (1988). *Psychiatric nursing*. Norwalk, CT: Addison-Wesley.

Zealberg, J. (1988). Care of patients with chronic mental illness: Letter to the editor. *New England Journal of Medicine, 318,* 1544.

IV

The Relationship Between Science and Practice

Commencing with Chapter 1, the relationships between science and scientific knowledge as well as the possibility of any application of scientific knowledge to practice were addressed within the purview of each specific school of thought. For this practice discipline, nursing, these relationships are both fundamental and critical to the structure of nursing knowledge and the process of nursing knowledge development.

In the three chapters comprising this section, very different relationships are proposed between science and practice. For Ann Bishop and John Scudder, the question is whether nursing can or will be a caring practice or an applied science. Hannah Dean explores several possible relationships: nursing as an academic/practice discipline, nursing as a science/technology, and nursing science/practice as a source of knowledge. Dean proposes that nursing is best served when the knowledge of the discipline emerges from a reciprocal, converging relationship among nursing theory, nursing science, and nursing practice. Finally, Luther Christman explores the relationship between science and nursing education and proposes that the essence of this relationship lies in the predictive nature of science in regard to professional recognition and success.

19

Applied Science, Practice, and Intervention Technology

ANNE H. BISHOP

JOHN R. SCUDDER, JR.

A fundamental issue in nursing concerns the very essence of nursing itself, namely, will nursing continue to be a caring practice, or will it become an applied science? The answer to this question depends on how applied science and practice are interpreted and on the relationships between them. We attempt to interpret and relate them in a way that will show that nursing is a caring practice that can be improved by use of applied science. First, we briefly consider the differences between interpreting nursing as an applied science and nursing as a practice (for a more extensive treatment of this difference, see Bishop & Scudder, 1990, 1991). Then we show, by critically appraising intervention technology, why nursing should be interpreted as a practice, not as an applied science, and how that interpretation allows the

263

incorporation of applied science into nursing practice without trans-
forming it into an applied science.

Practice and Applied Science

Nursing traditionally has called itself a practice. Even though the
meaning of practice was not usually articulated, referring to nursing as a
practice gave a certain identity to the nursing care given to patients.
Presumably nurses, in calling their profession a practice, had in mind
a meaning similar to that of the practice of medicine. Before the advent
of contemporary medical science, with its intervention technology, the
practice of medicine referred to traditional ways of caring for the well-
being of the ill or debilitated. Thus health care practice was traditionally not value neutral but positively attempted to foster the physical
and psychological well-being of persons. Therefore, although health
care professionals, and especially physicians, were inclined to wrap
themselves in the mantle of science, both medical and nursing practice
actually had a moral foundation. The moral sense of health care included not only care for the ill but also fostering good health. For this
reason, health care practice was actually more akin to practical wisdom
than to science or applied science.

The reason why nursing is better interpreted as a practice than as a
technology becomes more evident in light of the distinction Gadamer
(1976/1981), a leading authority on hermeneutics, makes between
practice and technology. He uses technology to mean what often is
designated as applied science. Designating applied science as technology is appropriate as technology refers primarily to a way of thinking
and doing rather than to things created for use. According to Gadamer,
technology is an application of scientific knowledge to the world so as
to control or intervene in some aspect of it. Of course, often the aim of
this control or intervention is to bring about something that is considered good. However, technology itself is neutral in the sense that it also
can be used to foster that which is considered evil. Also, in technology
the means used are separated from the ends sought. In contrast, a
practice seeks to bring about a certain good in ways that are integrally
related to the good sought. Thus the ways of a practice are integrally
related to the good it is designed to achieve, and its primary sense
concerns how that good is fostered in the world.

Gadamer's distinction between applied science and practice is help-ful in understanding nursing as a practice, but does it help us under-stand the discipline of nursing? The discipline of nursing is different from the practice of nursing. Unfortunately, nursing uses the same word to designate a practice and the systematic inquiry into the mean-ings and processes of that practice. For this reason, when someone uses the word nursing, it is difficult to discern whether they are talking about theories that attempt to clarify and articulate the meaning of practice or about the practice itself. This confusion further obscures the perennial difficult issue of the relation of theory to practice. Theoreti-cians who follow the applied science approach claim that this relation-ship is clear. Theory prescribes practice, but practitioners often complain that such theory distorts practice if, indeed, it has any relevance to practice at all.

The relationship of theory to practice is not a problem as Gadamer interprets theory. According to Gadamer (1976/1981), to the Greeks *theoria* meant "the eye disciplined enough to discern the visibly struc-tured order . . .of the world and of human society" (p. 69; for a more extensive treatment of how Gadamer's interpretation of practice re-lates to nursing, see Bishop & Scudder, 1990, pp. 67-78). Following the Greeks and Gadamer, such a theory of nursing would seek to disclose the meaning structures of nursing as it is practiced. For example, consider the meaning structure of the term "intervention." This term originated in medicine in the meaning structure of the cure of disease where it meant intervening in the natural development of a disease. Nurses adopted this term from medicine and used it vaguely to refer to what nurses do for, with, and to clients/patients. To designate all nursing care as intervention seems strange indeed. This odd way of speaking results from replacing a meaning structure of care with that of cure. When the meaning structure becomes care for the well-being of persons, it is the illness that intervenes in the person's well-being. As we will show later, a theory that imposes external meaning struc-tures from outside nursing, such as the use of intervention to designate all nursing care, is very different from one that is taken from nursing as practiced.

Some nursing scholars also have attempted to restructure nursing with systems of meaning taken from the behavioral sciences. The behavioral sciences grew out of the development of the social sciences that began in the latter part of the 19th century. Initially, the social sciences tended to copy the natural sciences. Those who followed this tendency to its logical conclusion changed the social sciences into the behavioral sciences. The tendency to reduce the social sciences to behavioral sciences led critics to charge that the behavioral sciences were eliminating the human from the study of social institutions and human relationships. Opposition to the reductive tendencies of the behavioral sciences fostered the development of the human sciences. The human sciences sought to develop a science that was appropriate to the study of man and of human affairs. One of the major concerns of the human sciences, especially in continental Europe, has been the development of the philosophy of practice. Practice has been neglected in the modern period due to the preoccupation with science and technology. Rather than focusing on knowledge and its use, practices concern the ways in which the good is accomplished in the world.

Stephen Strasser (1985), a Dutch phenomenologist, helps us understand how practice can be studied by contrasting it with scientific study. A science aims at discovery of the truth by using theories to make sense out of some aspect of the world and uses various methods, especially experimentation, to test the adequacy of that truth. In contrast, a practice fosters certain goods in the world. For example, political practice fosters effective social organization and justice. Health care, including nursing, fosters the physical and psychological well-being of persons. The adequacy of a practice is judged by how well it achieves the good at which it aims. Therefore, the discipline that studies a practice articulates ways that practice achieves its good. Strasser calls the disciplines that study practices the practical human sciences. Some practical human sciences that have specific names are political science, criminology, and jurisprudence. Some disciplines, such as education, medicine, and nursing, have the same name as the practice they study. However, regardless of whether or not these disciplines share the same name as the practice, their aim is not only to articulate the practice but also to improve the practice so that it can better achieve the good it is designed to foster.

Human science enlightens practitioners by disclosing the nature of practice, including possibilities for improved practice. Improving practice by realizing possibilities inherent within it keeps practices from merely being repetitions of traditional meanings and procedures. In fact, Alasdair MacIntyre (1984), a leading proponent of virtue ethics, contends that a practice that fails to develop by realizing possibilities is dead. In contrast to improvement through enlightened reform by practitioners, applied science seeks improvement from expert theoreticians who prescribe practice. If nursing were applied science, theory, tested by experimentation, would prescribe how nursing care is to be given. Thus what is at stake in determining the nature of the discipline is not merely how nursing should be studied but how nursing practice itself is constituted. The primary issue is the constitution of nursing itself, not the importance of applied science for nursing care. Any adequate study of contemporary nursing would need to recognize the importance of applied science in nursing practice, but there is an important difference between practices that use applied sciences and so-called "practices" that actually *are* applied sciences.

Although nursing often applies science, there are at least three reasons for believing that its fundamental constitution is that of a practice rather than that of an applied science. Nursing is a practice because (a) it is learned primarily through clinical experience, (b) it aims at particular care rather than uniform production, and (c) its primary sense is moral rather than theoretical.

First, practices are learned primarily through actual experience with and under the guidance of an expert practitioner. An applied science usually is not learned primarily through clinical experience. Mastering a science usually implies mastering a body of theory that designates the meaning of a predetermined portion of the world. When that theory is applied to practical ends, one has technology. The key to learning technology is first to learn the theory and then how to apply it. The how-to requires actual concrete instruction, but this instruction is very different from that required to learn a practice. The key to learning a practice is not primarily learning the theory and how to apply it but appropriating that practice by making it one's own, understanding its meaning, and employing it to achieve the moral good of the practice. The fact that nursing is learned primarily from clinical experience is a strong indication that it is a practice.

Second, technology follows a uniform process that prescribes the same techniques to produce the same result. For example, quality control in an automobile plant seeks one system that always produces the same product. Therefore, excellence in a technological system requires uniformity based on common techniques drawn from the same theory. Excellence in a practice comes not from impersonal uniformity but from personal excellence that results from appropriating the common practice in ways appropriate for the practitioner and to the persons cared for in their particular situations. For example, Benner (1984), drawing on Dreyfus and Dreyfus, has shown how the expert nurse is one who knows what needs to be done and how to do it without conscious reference to the theories and methodologies required of novice nurses. Expert veteran nurses work creatively within a web of meaning and therefore rarely follow a rigid, prescribed method. For example, a professor when asked how he liked his nurse during his brief stay in the hospital described her as a middle-aged nurse who cared for him rigidly, "according to the book." His colleagues in the nursing department knew immediately the name of the nurse because it is very unusual for veteran nurses to function in the same way that we expect novice nurses to function. We use this example to indicate how we ordinarily distinguish between a novice and an expert nurse. Novices generally slavishly follow a routine procedure given to them by others. In contrast, expert nurses master nursing practice by developing their own style of practice suited to their own particular way of caring and by fashioning their practice in ways appropriate to care for each particular patient in his or her situation. Rather than being a uniform process that produces the same product, nursing is a practice that is personally appropriated in ways that creatively foster the well-being of particular persons in certain situations.

Third, the dominant sense of practice is moral, whereas the dominant sense of technology is theoretical. Benner's (1984) exhaustive study of nursing competencies suggests that nursing is a practice with a dominant moral sense. It is significant that her study disclosed the moral sense of nursing even though it was not primarily designed to determine whether nursing had a moral sense. Unlike Benner's study, our study (Bishop & Scudder, 1990) of 40 practicing nurses specifically attempted to discern if nurses regarded the dominant sense of nursing as moral-personal or theoretical-technical. We asked them to describe the situation in which they were most fulfilled as a nurse. In every case but one, they described an experience that had a dominant moral-personal sense. This was true not only of nurses in community hospitals but also of those in a university medical center. The following description given by a nurse in a university medical center shows how even complex intervention technology can be incorporated into nursing care with a strong moral sense. This intensive care nurse described her patient who had undergone an aneurysm clipping as "a GCS5T, E4 M1,

VT [who] opened his eyes but [had] no movement and was trached"
(Bishop & Scudder, 1990, p. 99). It is obvious from this description that
this nurse worked in a highly technical situation. But she abandoned her
technological language when she expressed her feelings concerning
the outcome of her nursing care. "I can't describe the sensation I felt;
but to see him follow a command for the first time—moving his thumb
made me feel wonderful inside. All our diligent nursing care, position-
ing, ROM, stimulation, etc. was working and it felt good" (Bishop &
Scudder, 1990, pp. 99-100). The elation that came from seeing a thumb
move involved understanding a whole complex system of nursing
care. However, when she expressed her delight at the outcome of this
complex care it was given as an expression of personal elation evoked
by the improved condition of her patient. Significantly, this nurse said
that although she liked working with complex technology she would
not continue in nursing were it not for the fulfillment that came from
the moral sense of nursing.

Intervention Technology

The ease with which this nurse seems to have integrated applied
science into a caring practice should not blind us to the consequences
of nursing being constituted as an applied science rather than as a
practice. We attempt to show what is at stake in interpreting nursing
as an applied science, rather than as a practice, by critically appraising
intervention technology.

The first nurse critic of intervention medicine was Florence Nightingale. She actually opposed the theory of germs as the cause of disease
(Rosenberg, 1979). Although the theory of germs would explain why
fewer patients died in her clean and well-ventilated hospitals than in
other hospitals regardless of the physicians who practiced there, she
believed that she did not need that theory to account for the success of
her hospitals. She believed that nature rather than medicine healed.
The function of nursing was to establish the conditions necessary for
the body to heal itself (Nightingale, 1859/1946, p. 75). She reasoned
that, if the theory of germs was right, medical science would eventually
learn how to kill germs. Then health care would be focused on medical
intervention rather than on natural healing fostered by nursing care.

Actually, it was not until the mid 20th century that medical science
sufficiently developed intervention technology adequate to challenge

traditional practice. The new approach, although it often spoke of medicine as a science, was actually a technology in that it involved applying medical science to the curing of disease. Medical science was applied to intervene in the natural development of disease. These interventions were done with new drugs such as antibiotics and with radical new surgery that transformed and replaced body parts rather than merely repairing them.

The degree to which the interventionist view of medicine has formed our conceptions of medical and nursing practices is seen in the extensive and uncritical use of interventionist language by nurses and physicians. For example, the suggestion that nurses "involve family or significant others in the care plan" has been designated as an intervention for hopelessness (Carpenito, 1989, p. 440). How could this sound suggestion drawn from nursing practice logically be designated an intervention? This inappropriate use of intervention language in nursing care indicates the degree to which intervention technology has uncritically infiltrated into nursing. Intervention language originally came from medicine, where it meant intervening in the life history of the disease. For some reason, in both medicine and nursing it has come to mean whatever is done to, for, and with patients. So much is this so in nursing that Watson (1985) felt compelled to use the term "intervention" in discussing nursing practice even though she believed it to be inappropriate (p. 74). The use of medical language that implies an interventionist system of meaning has permeated other professions. Its use in education, according to Rose (1989, p. 209), not only has distorted education but actually has harmed students. We believe that this is also true of nursing. Intervention implies applying science to disease to kill it. If medicine is primarily intervention, then care is replaced by cure. Of course, intervention medicine is imperfect at present; consequently, there are patients with diseases who still require old-fashioned care, but according to the logic of intervention medicine, as medical science improves, this type of care will disappear. If cure becomes primary in health care, nurses would once again become the handmaidens of physicians. Physicians are the ones who apply science to the disease so as to cure it. However, physicians need assistants to help them care for patients as they are being cured. If cure becomes primary and care secondary, it follows that the curers, namely, physicians, would reserve their valuable time for cure, whereas carers, namely, nurses, would supervise recovery from disease and intervention. Thus this transformation of health care from care of persons to cure of disease would have serious implications for nursing. Besides reducing nursing to assisting physicians in cure, it would focus nursing on fighting disease rather than caring for the well-being of persons by fostering their health.

Before the advent of intervention technology, it was injury, illness, and debilitation that were understood to intervene in the lives of patients. Illness itself was experienced as intervention in accustomed and desired ways of living. The aim of health care was to restore the person to health by care. But contemporary intervention technology has changed the thrust of health care from restoring or promoting health to eradicating disease. If, however, the contemporary stress on health promotion continues to grow, it could initiate a movement away from interpreting health care as intervention and toward restoring it to the original meaning of fostering health through care.

Restoring health care to its original meaning does not imply diminishing the importance of intervention technology and cure in medicine. Anyone who has had an infection is thankful for antibiotics. The issue that concerns us here is not the importance of intervention technology but whether health care should be interpreted as intervention in disease or as fostering well-being or health. Interventions do, in fact, in many cases foster well-being, but often in so doing, they injure the body in ways that require nursing care.

When medical intervention is considered as just an important contribution to health care rather than its essence, then intervention technology will foster nursing that stresses care. Nursing care is needed not only because of illness or injury but because of what the medical interventions themselves do to the human body, as the following example illustrates. A nurse is caring for two patients, both of whom have been injured by knife wounds. The first wound was made by a direct straightforward stab that injured none of the vital organs. The second knife wound cut open the whole chest cavity and injured the heart beyond repair. The first wound was inflicted by a criminal who attacked a person who had resisted an attempted robbery. The second wound was inflicted by a surgeon who was performing a heart transplant. The first wound was inflicted to hurt, the second to help. In spite of malfeasant intent in the first wounding and beneficent intent in the second wounding, the second wound harmed the body far more than the first. The nurse who cares for both of these bodies will have to give much greater attention to the one injured by the surgeon's knife. One of the primary functions of contemporary nursing is to foster the healing of bodies that have suffered massive injury due to medical interventions. It is difficult to imagine greater interventions into the natural processes of the human body than cutting out a person's heart and replacing it with someone else's.

Heart transplant surgery and chemotherapy are dramatic examples of radical changes taking place in medical practice. Edmund Pellegrino (1985), president of the Kennedy Institute for the Study of Biomedical Ethics, contends that intervening in the natural history of disease through drug therapy and reconstructive surgery has greatly enhanced medicine's ability to cure. However, he fears that intervention technology is threatening the caring tradition of both the medical and the nursing practice. He contends that it is neither feasible nor desirable to return to the caring tradition of pre-intervention medicine. Instead, he contends that we need to interpret caring in a way that can incorporate intervention medicine into both the medical and the nursing practice.

Gadow (1985) attempted to interpret caring in a way that can incorporate medical intervention. She contends that such interventions challenge the caring tradition in at least two ways. The first is that intervention directs the center of one's experience to technological instruments and to the expert who controls them. In other words, one's health care comes under the control of machinery, chemicals, and the experts who prescribe and control them and thus control the patient's life. More important, she points out that technological intervention inclines us to think of the body itself as a machine. Care that takes into consideration technological intervention requires attending to the body object without reducing the person to the status of an object. In other words, nurses should care for patients by attending to the body object while relating to the patients as persons. Gadow claims that this can be done by the way in which we talk with and touch patients. Nurses should dialogically explore the meaning of illness and treatment with patients, rather than telling them objective statements of fact in the language of medical science. Also, nurses should touch patients empathically so as to communicate their care for them as fellow human beings. Medical intervention fosters instrumental touching that probes and manipulates the body impersonally as if the body of the nurse were an instrument and the body of the patient a machine. Although Gadow recognizes that instrumental touching is necessary in nursing care, she contends that empathic touching that brings nurse and patient into contact with each other as human beings confirms the humanity of both nurse and patient, even when attending to the body object.

The following example illustrates how nurses can care for the body object without reducing the person to the status of an object. "Joe" had outlived the prognosis for his type of cancer by at least 3 years. When he discussed his treatment for cancer, he constantly praised his nurse, "Beth," of whom he said, "She is on my team and she brought me through." Joe contrasted Beth with his physician, who he described as being very competent in intervention technology. His physician diagnosed and prescribed in impersonal language replete with technical and professional jargon. In contrast, Beth related to Joe primarily as a fellow human being, in that she talked with him and touched him as a person for whom she cared. Of course, she was technologically competent in administering the chemotherapy, in explaining his prescriptions to him, and in gaving directions on how to take them. She cheerfully responded when he called to ask how to lessen the pain, how to control the diarrhea, and how to alleviate the constipation, which often were more the consequence of treatment than illness. In short, although she was involved in administering the technological intervention, she gave the care that helped Joe bear the interventions. Her care helped the body heal and his spirit to cope with the consequences of intervention, but first and foremost, throughout the interventions she related to Joe as a fellow human being for whom she cared.

The story of Joe and Beth brings into focus two often obscured aspects of contemporary nursing care: first, that intervention technology increases the need for the care traditionally associated with nursing rather than decreasing it and, second, that this kind of care cannot be encompassed within nursing interpreted as applied science. However, applied science can be incorporated within nursing interpreted as the practice of care.

We have attempted to show what is at stake if nursing is restructured as an applied science by considering the example of Beth and Joe. Such examples are helpful to clarify meaning concretely. Joe's physician seems to be an intervention technologist for whom medical practice and care are anachronistic designations. In contrast, although Beth competently administered intervention technology, she was not primarily a technician but a nurse in a caring relationship with her patient. Note that caring here does not mean being personable and pleasant while structuring nursing as technological intervention. Care is a way of being with another person. In this case, that way of being is the care of the practice of nursing. Beth's personal appropriation of this practice made it possible for her to incorporate technical competency within the traditional practice of nursing care. An essential task for nursing in the years ahead is to incorporate technological intervention into the caring tradition so as to maintain and enhance the practice of fostering healing and health through caring relationships that affirm and enhance our shared humanity.

References

Benner, P. (1984). *From novice to expert: Excellence and power in clinical nursing practice.* Menlo Park, CA: Addison-Wesley.

Bishop, A. H., & Scudder, J. R., Jr. (1990). *The practical, moral, and personal sense of nursing: A phenomenological philosophy of practice.* Albany: State University of New York Press.

Bishop, A. H., & Scudder, J. R., Jr. (1991). *Nursing: The practice of caring.* New York: National League for Nursing.

Carpenito, L. J. (1989). *Nursing diagnosis: Application to clinical practice: Third edition 1989-1990.* Philadelphia: J. B. Lippincott.

Gadamer, H. G. (1981). *Reason in the age of science* (F. G. Lawrence, Trans.). Cambridge: MIT Press. (Original work published 1976)

Gadow, S. (1985). Nurse and patient: The caring relationship. In A. H. Bishop & J. R. Scudder, Jr. (Eds.), *Caring, curing, coping: Nurse, physician, patient relationships* (pp. 31-43). University: University of Alabama Press.

MacIntyre, A. (1984). *After virtue* (2nd ed.). Notre Dame, IN: University of Notre Dame Press.

Nightingale, F. (1946). *Notes on nursing.* Philadelphia: Edward Stern. (Original work published 1859)

Pellegrino, E. (1985). The caring ethic: The relation of physician to patient. In A. H. Bishop & J. R. Scudder, Jr. (Eds.), *Caring, curing, coping: Nurse, physician, patient relationships* (pp. 8-30). University: University of Alabama Press.

Rose, M. (1989). *Lives on the boundary.* New York: Penguin.

Rosenberg, C. E. (1979). Florence Nightingale on contagion: The hospital as moral universe. In C. E. Rosenberg (Ed.), *Healing and history* (pp. 116-136). New York: Dawson Science History Publications.

Strasser, S. (1985). *Understanding and explanation: Basic ideas concerning the humanity of the human sciences.* Pittsburgh, PA: Duquesne University Press.

Watson, J. (1985). *Nursing: Human science and human caring.* Norwalk, CT: Appleton-Century-Crofts.

20

Science and Practice

The Nature of Knowledge

HANNAH DEAN

Nursing's search for its professional identity has pervaded the professional literature over at least the past half century. This drive led to the development of master's and doctoral programs and increasingly sophisticated research activity. Nursing research progressed from occasional studies focused on nurses to well-developed programs of research that have built the body of knowledge in specific areas of client care. Examples of such programs are pain management, self-care practices, family health, women's health, and the care of low-birth-weight infants. The focus of this book, nursing's search for its scientific identity, is a natural extension of nursing's search for its professional identity.

Scientific efforts in nursing also have multiplied with the increasing number of persons qualified to serve as principal investigators. The development of nursing science initially was influenced by the methods and worldview of the various related fields in which nurses originally sought doctoral degrees: education, anthropology, psychology, sociology, and physiology. Also, over the past 20 years, doctoral programs in nursing have proliferated. As a result, a cadre developed of doctorally prepared nurses whose entire educational experience occurred in the context of nursing as the primary discipline.

The purpose of this chapter is to explore the relationship among beliefs about science and the nature of scientific inquiry and practice, especially as this relationship exists in professional disciplines such as nursing. The chapter examines several dialectics that affect the relationship: namely, nursing as an academic discipline/nursing as a practice discipline, nursing as a science/nursing as a technology, and nursing science as a source of knowledge/nursing practice as a source of knowledge. Currently, nursing theory, nursing research, and nursing practice exist largely as separate entities. The basic proposition of this chapter is that nursing's ability to meet its obligations to society is at its best when the knowledge of the discipline emerges from a reciprocal, converging relationship between nursing theory, nursing science, and nursing practice and that both unity and diversity of thought lead to knowledge development.

Nursing as an Academic Discipline/ Nursing as a Practice Discipline

In the late 1940s and early 1950s, preparation of nurses shifted from an apprenticeship training model to a college-based academic model. Formerly, education and practice were closely linked, with education heavily influenced by practice. In its effort to establish itself as a profession, nursing eschewed the apprenticeship model and embraced the academic model. The gradual change separated nursing as an academic discipline from nursing as a practice discipline (Dean & Lee, 1992).

Nurses involved in the academic arena adhere to the cultural expectations of that environment. Some of these nurses focus on conceptual models or theoretical formulations of the discipline as a way to organize curricula and give them coherence or structure. Others focus on scientific productivity and strive to compete/survive in an environment that values research and publication as primary measures of performance. Still other academic-based nurses respond to the pressure to produce sufficient numbers of practitioners, teaching large numbers of students to function in a work environment. Whatever the academic setting, nursing faculty strive to develop and transmit the body of knowledge and the worldview that constitute their image of nursing. Usually, these faculty have limited contact with nursing as a practice discipline. For some, the contact consists of supervision of students in clinical settings; for others, there may be no direct contact with the practice discipline except as consumers of health care services.

Nurses in the practice arena adhere to the cultural expectations of an altogether different environment. Nurses in clinical practice respond to increasingly difficult nursing practice and delivery problems (Aiken, 1982). Benner's (1984) work documents the wide range of responsibilities incumbent on nurses in clinical practice—from providing comfort measures to managing pain to responding to life-threatening emergencies. Nursing as a practice discipline faces challenges posed by the changes in care delivery systems. For example, the decrease in length of stay reduces the time available for preoperative teaching and discharge planning. The shift to ambulatory care demands politically astute nurses who can make the case for and deliver nursing care outside the hospital setting. Practicing nurses also develop and transmit a body of knowledge and a worldview that constitute their image of nursing. This image may or may not be consistent with the image held by nurses in the academic arena. Usually, these nurses have limited or no contact with nursing as an academic discipline. Some may interact with faculty who are with students on their units; others have no contact at all. Some may read scholarly journals and research-based literature; others read practice-based journals that make no pretense at scholarship; still others read not at all.

Aiken (1982) sounded an alarm when she said, "One factor that has contributed significantly to the worsening employment conditions in hospitals has been the gradual separation between nurses who educate students and those who practice nursing. . . . A large proportion [of nurses with advanced preparation] . . . have remained in academic institutions rather than put their increased knowledge and skills into use in practice settings" (p. 92). The same issue applies to nurses who engage in the practice of research. The majority are academically based, thus separating them from practice settings and nurses in clinical practice. The separation between the knowledge producers (scientists), knowledge users (practitioners), and knowledge transmitters (educators) creates disparity, dissonance, and disunity that is at once dangerous and advantageous. The danger lies in the potential for professional divisiveness. The advantage is the growth made possible by the increasing knowledge brought to bear by the scientists, practitioners, and educators, each striving for new knowledge in their own realms.

Nursing as a Science/Nursing as a Technology or an Art

Harding (1991) distinguishes between the sciences and their technologies. She says, "Science and technology can be discrete not because science is autonomous from technology (for it never is) but because technological innovation is sometimes autonomous from science—but 'sometimes' is not always" (p. 242). The use of the word technology will rankle those who distinguish between professional and technical nursing. Perhaps Brink's (1993) distinction between science and art is more acceptable. In either case, the focus of this book is nursing's search for its scientific identity, and this chapter's specific focus is the relationship between science and practice (technology or art).

According to Harding's (1991) thesis, nursing science is inextricably related to nursing technology (practice or art), but nursing technology is not necessarily similarly linked to nursing science. Benner (1984) points to the lack of commitment to nursing science in the technology arena as a barrier to retention of expert clinicians at the bedside. The nursing research utilization literature reflects this issue in articles that examine the barriers to the use of nursing research (Fawcett, 1984; Ferrell, Grant, & Rhiner, 1990; Funk, Champagne, Wiese, & Tornquist, 1991; Gennaro & Vessey, 1991). In spite of Harding's (1991) perspective, each of these authors makes the case that research-based practice is vital to professional practice in nursing.

NURSING SCIENCE

What constitutes nursing science? Science generated by other disciplines affects nursing practice, and nursing science affects other disciplines. Nursing technology relies on scientific knowledge generated in other disciplines such as psychology, sociology, and physics (Gennaro & Vessey, 1991). Conversely, scientific knowledge generated by nurse scientists such as Benoliel in the area of death and dying and Johnson in the area of patient education (both cited in Farrell et al., 1990) has had significant impact on patient care in general, not only on care delivered by nurses. In a speech at the UCLA School of Nursing, Donaldson (1990) proposed that nursing science is misnamed, that it is more properly the study of human responses to actual or potential health problems; thus the science would be distinct from the technology. Some express concern that a large number of nurse scientists educated in related disciplines such as psychology or physiology may identify with nursing technology so weakly that they do not "value or even recognize nursing's disciplinary matrix and/or may not be interested in studying the phenomena with which nurses are concerned" (Riegel et al., 1992). The basic premise underlying this chapter is that the knowledge of the discipline emerges from a reciprocal relationship between nursing theory, nursing science, and nursing practice, that nursing's ability to meet its obligations to society is best when the three converge (Adam, 1992). However, knowledge generated either by science or through practice belongs in the public domain and is available to whoever may find it useful.

Riegel et al. (1992) indicate that nursing science seems to be in search of an appropriate, existing philosophy of science. The adoption of such a philosophy would result in consequent adoption of related, compatible epistemologies (Lindeman, 1984; Smith, 1984). Riegel et al. (1992) analyze the influence of four major schools of thought: logical positivism and the paradigmatic, evolutionary, and feminist schools. They contend that none of the approaches sufficiently reflects the complexity and richness of nursing. They propose a philosophy for practice disciplines, which is described in detail in another chapter in this book. Briefly, they insist that knowledge development in a practice discipline "must have clinical relevance to be useful to the technicians and professionals in clinical practice and to society in general" (p. 118). Research produces knowledge in the discipline only as it is consistent with the matrix of the discipline, that is, the structure, tradition, values, and beliefs of the discipline. As Fawcett (1984) says, "In the final analysis the most important consideration is the contribution of the findings of any one study to nursing knowledge" (p. 62).

NURSING PRACTICE

Nursing practice is grounded in values, beliefs, and practices including caring, health promotion, nurturing, involvement, helping people deal with their reality, and recognizing nonlinear multiple causes and the importance of context. These values and beliefs are articulated eloquently by feminist scholars (Belenky, Clinchy, Goldberger, & Tarule, 1986; Harding, 1991) and nursing scholars (Benner, 1984; Phillips, 1992; Roach, 1992). Other values, beliefs, and practices such as curing, controlling, distance, and searching for linear causality irrespective of context are more characteristic of male-dominated disciplines and male-dominated approaches to science. Harding (1991) states,

> Metaphors and models that stress context rather than isolated traits and behaviors, interactive rather than linear relations, and democratic rather than authoritarian models of order in both research and nature . . . have been associated with womanliness; their use can be thought of as infusing values arising from women's lives into scientific practices and outcomes. (p. 301)

Benner's (1984) analysis of the phenomenon of *caring* as central to excellent nursing practice underscores this feminist value. Benner (1984) urges scholarly inquiry as she recognizes the challenges that caring presents. Her description points to the need for a philosophy of science consistent with the demands of such inquiry:

> Nursing is a human science, conducted by self-interpreting subjects (researchers) who are studying self-interpreting subjects (participants) who *both* may change as a result of an investigation. . . . Caring cannot be controlled or coerced; it can only be understood and facilitated. Caring is embedded in personal and cultural meanings and commitments. . . . Therefore, the strategies for studying it must take into account meanings and commitments. (p. 171)

She contends that we cannot rely solely on the natural science model of quantitative, experimental approaches.

Phillips (1992) adds another dimension to the nature of nursing practice; he states that "the core of nursing lies in the *wholeness* of human beings" (p. 49). In my own experience as a nurse, I came to the clearest existential realization of my identity as a nurse when I was involved in hospice care. Two specific instances come to mind: The first reflects the wholeness of human beings; the second illustrates nursing's focus on caring. The first was at an international and multidisciplinary meeting of cancer researchers and providers. The meeting was dominated by physicians and basic scientists with a few nurses, social workers, and patient education specialists. The enormous hall of commercial exhibitors included a number of publishers with books related to cancer. Among the collection of books offered, I found none about the human experience of cancer and none about whole beings; every book focused on parts of beings (human and otherwise), many at the cellular level.

The second sharp memory involved a patient who had been referred to hospice care by his physician. The elderly patient and his wife understood that he was terminally ill and wanted him to die at home. When I asked the physician for the medical orders necessary to permit third-party payment of the care to be provided, he said, "I have no idea what he needs. You decide, write the orders, and I'll sign them." The physician recognized that the patient's needs for caring were outside the realm of his expertise of curing. The frustration for me was that my expertise in caring was unacceptable to the third-party payor unless it was presented with the physician's signature, reflecting the dominance of the medical model.

It is the nature of nursing practice to focus on wholeness rather than parts, on caring rather than curing, on helping patients and families cope with their reality rather than trying to control or alter their reality, on helping patients and families care for themselves to the extent possible rather than on treating them, and on the primacy of interpersonal dynamics of the nurse patient relationship rather than on the provider as authority. Roach (1992) says, "The focal points of human care, human person, and person-in-relation (the human community), along with a duty to care, mark the unifying elements and the ground for 'first causes' or 'first principles' in nursing" (p. 42).

In the past, these characteristics have impeded nursing science and practice and recognition of the profession's contributions because of the preeminence of male-dominated models. Economic support for research and practice has favored strongly the biomedical models. In the context of current changes in the health care delivery system, the knowledge and skills of nursing's disciplinary matrix are likely to have increasing support. The increasing focus on quality of life as an outcome measure beyond the traditional measures of mortality and morbidity provides evidence of this shift.

Nursing Science and Nursing Practice as Sources of Knowledge

The push for research-based practice runs the risk of idealizing nursing research and denigrating nursing practice. Both nursing scientists and nursing practitioners (technologists, artists) need to have a healthy respect for their own and each other's strengths and weaknesses. The knowledge gained from both nursing research and practice is valuable and flawed. Neither research knowledge nor practice knowledge alone is sufficient.

In her classic article, Carper (1978) identifies four fundamental patterns of knowing: empirics, aesthetics, personal, and ethics. In this schema, science (empirics) takes its place among other, equally important sources of knowledge. Holm and Llewellyn (1986) likewise identify multiple types of inquiry, including logical reasoning, experience, tradition, custom, precedent, habit, authority, trial and error, and research, both basic and applied. Belenky et al. (1986) distinguish women's ways of knowing from men's ways of knowing. They contend that "all knowledge is constructed" and "that the knower is an intimate part of the known" (p. 137).

Carper (1992) synthesizes her model and the work of Jacobs-Kramer and Chinn (cited in Carper, 1992) by summarizing the three dimensions of their model (creation, expression, and assessment) with her four patterns of knowing. Table 20.1 summarizes Carper's synthesis: The rows summarize the ways that knowledge is created, expressed, and assessed; the columns are the ways of knowing. Carper's synthesis provides a framework for evaluating and valuing a range of sources of knowledge in a practice discipline.

Holm and Llewellyn (1986) acknowledge a variety of sources of knowledge. However, the tone of their work reflects a strong influence from what Guba (1990) would call positivism and what is called traditional thought or the received view in a section of this book. That is to say, they state that the purpose of research is to discover the *truths*

TABLE 20.1   A Model for the Creation, Expression, and Assessment of the
Patterns of Knowing

	Empirical	Ethical	Personal	Esthetic
Creation	Research methods for: describing, explaining, predicting	Processes for extending knowledge: valuing, clarifying, advocating	Encountering, focusing on, realizing self and others	Engaging, interpreting, envisioning
Expression	Understanding due to: facts, models, theories, descriptions	Codes, moral rules, decision making	Authentic and disclosed self, I-Me congruity	Art-act
Assessment	What does this represent? How is it representative?	Is this right? Is this just? Is this good?	Do I know what to do? Do I do what I know?	What does this mean?
Process/ Context for addressing assessment questions	Replication	Dialogue	Response reflection	Interpretation of meaning
Credibility index	Validity	Justness (caring, connection)	Congruity	Consensus

SOURCE: Adapted from Carper 1992, p. 78-79.

of the discipline (emphasis added). They use words like explain, predict, and control. In their discussion of types of inquiry, they focus primarily on the relationship between theory and research, giving only lip service to practice—this in spite of the title of their book, *Nursing Research for Nursing Practice.*

In contrast to Holm and Llewellyn, Belenky et al. (1986) describe "constructed knowledge" and quote one of their subjects:

In science you don't really want to say that something's true. You realize that you're dealing with a model. Our models are always simpler than the real world. The real world is more complex that anything we can create. We're simplifying everything so that we can work with it, but the thing is really more complex. When you try to describe things, you're leaving the truth because you're oversimplifying. (p. 138)

In this view of knowledge, explanation, prediction, and control are recognized as relative to the knower. Other explanations and predictions are possible, and control is virtually impossible.

Nursing the academic discipline, nursing the practice discipline, nursing science, and nursing technology all contribute to nursing knowledge. The challenge for all participants is to respect and value a variety of ways of knowing and a variety of approaches to science. A single approach or a limited range of approaches is unlikely to yield the depth of knowledge required to provide excellent nursing care. Representative George E. Brown, Jr. (D-California), in an op-ed article (Brown, 1992), calls for a new contract with the scientific community measuring the value of research in terms of its use. He suggests that we need systems to incorporate what we know for the benefit of society. A number of questions are raised by these points of view: Who is responsible for the generation of knowledge? Who is responsible for identifying research agenda? Who is responsible for the use of research? Are researchers responsible? Are practitioners (technologists, artists) responsible? What about theoreticians? What about teachers, policymakers, and administrators? Aren't all responsible, individually and in concert?

Nursing Theory, Nursing Research, and Nursing Practice as Separate and Interrelated Exercises

In the real world, in nursing as it is contemplated, researched, practiced, taught, organized, regulated, and administered, there is separation and overlap among these various activities. Nursing theorists operate in their world as do nursing scientists, nursing practitioners (technologists, artists), and nursing administrators in theirs. Nurse theorists and nurse scientists may be educators or educational administrators also. Some nursing research is theory based; most curricula are organized around a conceptual framework, if not a theory, to meet accreditation criteria; and nursing service is beginning to incorporate research into procedures to meet accreditation criteria. The professional literature is replete with admonitions that research must be theory based, that curricula must be theory based, that practice must be research based, that faculty must be clinically competent, and that education and service must reach rapprochement at the least. The signs and symptoms of separation of theory, science, and practice clearly are evident as are the overlaps. The great challenge facing a practice discipline, such as nursing, is to strain against the edges of growth and development while maintaining a unity of purpose in meeting the needs of society, which is, after all, the reason for the existence of practice disciplines.

Nursing theories emerged as the discipline evolved from the apprenticeship model of training to the university- and college-based model of education. Nursing educators strived to educate students to know *why* as well as to know *how*. The primary impetus for theory development derived from educators rather than from clinicians. Nursing theories helped faculties organize and structure knowledge. As students taught in theory-based programs completed their course work and entered practice settings, the effect of nursing theory began to be visible in practice to a limited extent. The adoption of a specific theoretical framework for use in a clinical setting depends on the commitment to that framework by nurses at all levels of the hierarchy. Diversity among clinicians renders consensus difficult to achieve. Individual clinicians may adhere to a theoretical framework to guide their own practice; however, the full impact of that approach is unlikely to be felt in patient care because of the large number of nursing personnel involved in the care of any one patient.

The two frameworks most commonly seen in clinical settings—nursing process and nursing diagnosis—are atheoretic. Nagle and Mitchell (1991) distinguish between the totality paradigm and the simultaneity paradigm. In their description, the nursing process and nursing diagnosis derive from the totality paradigm, represented by logical empiricism and an objective, reductionist point of view. They contend that the totality paradigm is inconsistent with nursing's caring, interactionist, holistic, nurturing focus. Models consistent with the simultaneity paradigm and that focus on caring, interaction, holism, and nurturing find support among theoreticians and educators but seldom are seen as foundations of practice in clinical settings. The dominance of the totality paradigm as opposed to the simultaneity paradigm probably relates to the male-dominated majority culture (Belenky et al., 1986).

Nursing research primarily emanates from university schools of nursing. The questions addressed, the methods chosen, and the samples selected are influenced by the context in which research is conducted. The expectations and limitations imposed by the context affect the product. Most of the major university schools of nursing exist in settings that also support schools of medicine; thus nurse researchers compete with physicians for research subjects and access to resources. Often, the associated clinical settings are organized primarily in support of the education and research efforts of physicians, with other health care professional schools adapting to rather than controlling the environment.

Generally, nurse theorists and nurse researchers have limited clinical involvement. The demands on their time and the geographic diversity of the placement of undergraduate and graduate students restrict their ability to develop strong relationships with clinically based nurses.

The majority of *nurses in practice* have little or no direct contact with nurse theorists or nurse researchers. More than 50% were educated in associate degree or diploma schools of nursing, where the primary goal was to teach large numbers of students to function in a work environment. Neither theory nor research enjoys a prominent position in the education or practice of these nurses. Their support of and appreciation for nursing theory and research is limited as is their ability to link theory, practice, and research.

The separation of nursing theorists, nursing researchers, and nursing practitioners from one another results from the context in which each operates. Each group responds to the demands of the environment in which it functions. Although much change has occurred, as witnessed by the growth of the number of doctoral programs in nursing in the past 25 years, still much remains to be accomplished in improving patient care and establishing the role of nursing in achieving desirable patient outcomes.

Proposed: A Three-Way
Collaborative Model

The separation of nursing theory, nursing research, and nursing practice limits knowledge development and constrains nursing's ability to meet its obligations to society as a practice discipline. Knowledge develops and is used most effectively when nursing theory, research, and practice converge.

A further effect of the separation of nursing theorists, researchers, and practitioners is the dilution of power and the weakening of influence. Most research use models identify nursing practitioners as users

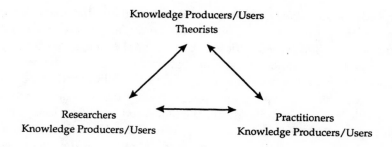

FIGURE 20.1. Three-way exchange model
SOURCE: Adapted from Boggs (1992, p. 37).

or consumers of research (Rempusheski, 1991). Boggs (1992) proposes a three-way exchange model of knowledge development and use. I have adapted the model to illustrate an alternate relationship among theorists, researchers, and practitioners I think is necessary for further development of the science and practice of nursing. In the three-way exchange model, all three parties are seen as knowledge producers and knowledge users. Figure 20.1 illustrates the three-way exchange model.

Conceiving knowledge production and use in this manner gives equal footing to all participants. It recognizes the mutuality necessary for the development of knowledge and eliminates elitist-peasant polarities among the players. The three-way exchange model places the responsibility for knowledge production and use equally on all parties and requires collaborative exchange. This approach has the potential for establishing creative coalitions that will address significant clinical issues in carefully designed studies based in clinically relevant theoretical frameworks.

Fawcett and Downs (1986) identify seven criteria to evaluate the relationship between theory and research. One of these, "Is pragmatic adequacy evident?," emphasizes the feasibility of innovative actions, the legal authority for the practitioner to carry out the innovation, and the congruence of the innovative actions with client expectations. This criterion coupled with their first criterion of significance to the discipline lends support to the value of the proposed adaptation of the three-way exchange model. Others (Mercer, 1984; Nail, 1990) emphasize the importance of researcher-clinician collaboration but fail to include theoreticians in the collaboration. I contend that all three major categories of players must operate collaboratively for the discipline to successfully find its scientific and professional practice identity.

Paradoxically, although the proposed model in this chapter demands unity of approach among theorist, researcher, and practitioner as they work together to create knowledge, diversity remains necessary and valuable in a professional discipline (Kim, 1983). Boggs (1992) distinguishes professionals from technicians on the basis of the availability of models into which the professional conceptualizes the client's concerns. In contrast to Kuhn's (1970) position that mature sciences work from a single dominant paradigm, it seems to me that the nature of nursing as a caring, holistic, human science requires multiple models, multiple epistemologies, and multiple approaches to clinical problems. Laudan's (1981) problem-solving approach to scientific progress maintains that the dialectical struggle between competing approaches leads to improvement and refinement based on the criticisms that emerge from the confrontation.

Summary

Nursing's search for its scientific identity is inextricably linked to its search for its professional identity. Professional education in nursing developed in direct contrast to the previous apprenticeship training model. Research productivity developed in the context of university-based professional education. The evolution of nursing research was influenced by the cadre of doctorally prepared nurses, first with doctorates in other fields and now with doctorates in nursing. Locating nursing education in colleges and universities served the development of the academic discipline but created a rift between the academic discipline and the practice discipline. Nursing theorists and nursing researchers primarily operate in the academic context separated from nursing practitioners in clinical settings.

Professional disciplines owe their existence to their mandate to serve society through their special knowledge and skills. Nursing, a predominantly female profession, is characterized by values, beliefs, and practices ordinarily associated with womanliness: namely, caring, health promotion, nurturing, involvement, helping people deal with their reality, and recognizing nonlinear multiple causes and the importance of context. The position of nursing as a health care profession is affected by the dominance of the male-oriented values that character-ize medicine as a profession: namely, curing, controlling, distance, and searching for linear causality irrespective of context.

Nursing knowledge develops most effectively in a three-way exchange among nursing theorists, nursing researchers, and nursing practitioners. This model of collaborative exchange identifies all participants as producers and users of knowledge. It emphasizes the equality of the importance of the contributions of the various players and requires communication and collaboration in the creation of knowledge. Diver-sity and competing theories or schools of thought can and should con-tinue to stimulate growth and development in the profession.

References

Adam, E. (1992). Contemporary conceptualizations of nursing: Philosophy or science? In J. F. Kikuchi & H. Simmons (Eds.), *Philosophic inquiry in nursing* (pp. 55-63). Newbury Park, CA: Sage.

Aiken, L. H. (Ed.). (1982). *Nursing in the 1980's: Crises, opportunities, challenges*. Philadel-phia: J. B. Lippincott.

Belenky, M. F., Clinchy, B. M., Goldberger, N. R., & Tarule, J. M. (1986). *Women's ways of knowing: The development of self, voice, and mind*. New York: Basic Books.

Benner, P. (1984). *From novice to expert: Excellence and power in clinical nursing practice*. Menlo Park, CA: Addison-Wesley.

Boggs, J. P. (1992). Implicit models of social knowledge use. *Knowledge, 14*(1), 29-62. .

Brink, P. J. (1993). The art and science of nursing. *Western Journal of Nursing Research, 15*(2), 145-147.

Brown, G. E. (1992, September 8). It's down to the last blank check. *Los Angeles Times,* op-ed section.

Carper, B. A. (1978). Fundamental patterns of knowing in nursing. *Advances in Nursing Science, 1,* 13-23.

Carper, B. A. (1992). Philosophical inquiry in nursing: An application. In J. F. Kikuchi & H. Simmons (Eds.), *Philosophic inquiry in nursing* (pp. 71-80). Newbury Park, CA: Sage.

Dean, H. E., & Lee, J. L. (1992, October). *Service and practice in partnership*. Paper presented at the annual meeting of the American Academy of Nursing, St. Louis.

Donaldson, S. K. (1990). *Building a research program: Credibility and diversity*. Speech delivered at the School of Nursing, University of California, Los Angeles.

Fawcett, J. (1984). Another look at utilization of nursing research. *Image, 16*(2), 59-62.

Fawcett, J., & Downs, F. S. (1986). *The relationship of theory and research*. Norwalk, CT: Appleton-Century-Crofts.

Ferrell, B. R., Grant, M. M., & Rhiner, M. (1990). Bridging the gap between research and practice. *Oncology Nursing Forum, 17*(3), 447-448.

Funk, S. G., Champagne, M. T., Wiese, R. A., & Tornquist, E. M. (1991). Barriers to using research findings in practice: The clinician's perspective. *Applied Nursing Research, 4*(2), 90-95.

Gennaro, S., & Vessey, J. (1991). Making practice perfect. *Nursing Research, 40*(5), 259.

Guba, E. C. (1990). The alternative paradigm dialogue. In E. C. Guba (Ed.), *The paradigm dialogue* (pp. 17-27). Newbury Park, CA: Sage.

Harding, S. (1991). *Whose science? Whose knowledge?* Ithaca, NY: Cornell University Press.

Holm, K., & Llewellyn, J. G. (1986). *Nursing research for nursing practice.* Philadelphia: W. B. Saunders.

Kim, H. S. (1983). *The nature of theoretical thinking in nursing.* Norwalk, CT: Appleton-Century-Crofts.

Kuhn, T. S. (1970). *The structure of scientific revolutions* (2nd ed.). Chicago: University of Chicago Press.

Laudan, L. (1981). A problem-solving approach to scientific progress. In L. Hacking (Ed.), *Scientific revolutions* (pp. 144-155). Oxford: Oxford University Press.

Lindeman, C. A. (1984). Dissemination of nursing research. *Image, 16*(2), 57-58.

Mercer, R. T. (1984). Nursing research: The bridge to excellence in practice. *Image, 16*(2), 47-51.

Nagle, L. M., & Mitchell, G. J. (1991). Theoretic diversity: Evolving paradigmatic issues in research and practice. *Advances in Nursing Science, 14*(1), 17-25.

Nail, L. M. (1990). Involving clinicians in research. *Oncology Nursing Forum, 17*(4), 621-623.

Phillips, J. R. (1992). The aim of philosophical inquiry in nursing: Unity or diversity of thought? In J. F. Kikuchi & H. Simmons (Eds.), *Philosophic inquiry in nursing* (pp. 45-50). Newbury Park, CA: Sage.

Rempusheski, V. F. (1991). Using art and science to change practice. *Applied Nursing Research, 4*(2), 96-98.

Riegel, B., Omery, A., Calvillo, E., Elsayed, N. G., Lee, P., Shuler, P., & Siegal, B. E. (1992). Moving beyond: A generative philosophy of science. *Image, 24*(2), 115-120.

Roach, M. S., Sr. (1992). The aim of philosophical inquiry in nursing: Unity or diversity of thought? In J. F. Kikuchi & H. Simmons (Eds.), *Philosophic inquiry in nursing* (pp. 38-44). Newbury Park, CA: Sage.

Smith, M. C. (1984). Research methodology. *Image, 16*(2), 42-46.

21

Science as the Predictor of Professional Recognition and Success

LUTHER CHRISTMAN

Clinical nursing practice is the application of science to eliminate or mitigate the physical and emotional problems of patients. To do this endeavor effectively requires nurses to have a broad general science base in the biophysical and behavioral sciences plus an in-depth scientific knowledge in the specialty area of practice. But what is the science that nurses are to integrate with their practice knowledge? Is it the science of empiricists or the science of postmodernists?

For many nurses, to answer this question they must first understand scientific knowledge. And to understand scientific knowledge they need to examine closely how scientists in general are educated. Traditionally, the prime focus in preparing scientists is on obtaining a very strong body of knowledge in the main area of concentration and minor preparation in related areas. Courses in the philosophy of science that

291

enable scientists to formulate scientific inquiry and a reasonable amount of research methods courses, which help fashion the question to be addressed in a research format congruent with the scientific undertaking, are also part of the educational process.

This mode of preparation at the doctoral level for scientists is often at variance with the doctorate preparation of nurses, the difference being the focus of content. In many nursing doctoral programs, advanced clinical and scientific preparation is downplayed, and a plethora of research methods courses and functional courses are the centerpieces of the various curricula. Imagine, for a moment, how few breakthroughs would occur in physics, biochemistry, sociology, psychology, or any of the sciences if the respective researchers did not have the strong content underpinnings to be able to ask the pertinent questions that enable steady (and in some cases startling) accomplishments.

An anecdote may help to illustrate this point. I was invited to speak at a university offering a doctoral in nursing. After the session ended, a nurse who had just completed all her doctoral preparation sought my attention. She expressed her enthusiasm about becoming a researcher. She then stated, "Now that I have taken all these many research courses all I have to do is find a problem that fits them." I replied, "That is not the usual approach to research. Research is asking the right question—a question in clinical practice that will improve the care of patients." She looked somewhat startled and said, "How come not even one faculty member explained that to me during my doctoral work?" I did not comment, but I thought it may have been because the faculty members themselves had been prepared with only a minimal amount of clinical and scientific content. Research courses in themselves are not a powerful tool if the needed content to conceptualize the fitness of the questions is absent.

One way of visualizing the scientific preparation of the future is to have a goodly number of nurses prepared at the combined doctoral level (D.N.Sc.-Ph.D.). This format then becomes the linchpin for focusing the body of needed science on patient care and at the same time feeding back from the clinical areas the needed scientific enterprises that would enrich and facilitate patient care.

The sciences involved in each practice area should complement and supplement each other. For instance, psychiatric nurses should concentrate on sociology, anthropology, psychology, neuroendocrinology, neurophysiology, and neuroanatomy. Community health nurses should have substantial preparation in general physiology, general anatomy, biochemistry, epidemiology, microbiology, anthropology, sociology, and psychology. Medical nurses should pursue basic science content from general physiology, exercise physiology (and physiology relevant to the selected subspecialty), biochemistry, microbiology, and psychology. Content from anthropology and sociology would enable discharge planning to be more comprehensive and accurate. The recruitment of scientists at the Ph.D. level into clinical nursing programs is another possibility to enlarge the critical mass of nurses prepared at this level. This in turn would accelerate the dissemination of science among nurses. The question remains, however, how the inevitable conflict between the divergent philosophies of these sciences and the philosophy of nursing will be resolved?

The possibility of preparation in two applied sciences offers another interesting pathway. Psychiatric nurses could pair a clinical doctorate in psychiatric nursing with a doctorate in clinical psychology. The clinical power from this approach is obvious. To gain a cluster of practitioners in this area might be useful to stimulate some clinical psychologists also to obtain a doctorate in psychiatric nursing. The same concepts could be used in biomedical engineering, with dual preparation starting from nurses or from engineers. An examination of biomedical research often shows the collaboration of physicians to enhance and facilitate research efforts that are advantageous to patient care. The addition of nurses to research of this type could produce new insights and increase the usefulness of this form of inquiry relevant to patient care. All the examples stated above have the potential for greatly raising the level of visibility and recognition of nurses. That is, of course, if the beliefs regarding science are congruent.

In this proposed route of preparation, it is presumed that all specialization will be at the doctoral level. Specialization at the master's level is not a realistic goal given the expanded knowledge system. Using the above as a general guide, one can go through all the areas of nursing practice and attach the sciences most useful to effectuate practice in each specific area. Although the depth and complexity of the mix of sciences will vary for each area (and within areas), they should be clustered according to the clinical practice area by priority of need. Nurses must decide whether this or a more creative approach will enable them to remain competent and needed in a cybernated system. Not to act may mean that the word technical will replace the word professional when referring to nurses. Will nurses use the method and content of science to transform the profession to a truly professional status? If so, which kind of science will it be? That continues to be nursing's critical question.

Epilogue

The Journey Continues

At this point, it is important to reassess where the ideas presented in this book have led us. In the Preface, we identified our belief that a plurality of philosophies may be necessary to reflect the many facets of nursing science, that no one view may be sufficient to embrace or drive nursing knowledge in all of its diversity. It is time to question whether this belief can still be supported. Further, if such a belief can be supported, can there be any unity in nursing science?

More than any other content presented, the application chapters support the ongoing need for diversity in belief systems, for it is only through that diversity that the discipline of nursing will be able to support knowledge development, scientific knowledge development in particular. The application content ranged from the further development of a philosophy of science for the discipline of nursing (Chapter 5) to the presentation of a clinical research study that had its method of inquiry firmly founded in a particular view of scientific method and knowledge (Chapter 12). Each of these contributions adds its own unique perspective to the totality that is this discipline nursing. Each of these contributions is founded within a unique school of thought. To deny

295

one of these belief systems at the expense of another is to deny a specific and unique contribution to our discipline.

We believe that such a denial would have a catastrophic effect on the continuing development of nursing knowledge. It would be as if on our journey through the terrain that is nursing we tried to climb a mountain with only one rope. Despite such a limitation, we might be able to scale a significant portion of the peak. Certainly, the empiricist and pragmatic terrains have contributed greatly to the development of nursing science; yet, as those proponents of alternative belief systems have identified, there are significant parts of the mountain that cannot be traversed if we are limited to a single rope. Thus many significant ideas would be rejected as directions in knowledge development for the discipline if empiricism were the only legitimate school of thought driving knowledge development.

Rather, it seems that we need to be open to diverse schools of thought. We must acknowledge the contributions that the empiricist belief system make possible. But as Gayle Page indicated, we may never scale the pain peak; we may never resolve the pain questions in science until we recognize the biases and potential for oppression that can present themselves within the context of the traditional belief systems of science and scientific knowledge.

If such diversity of belief is tolerated in our discipline, will the inevitable outcome be a lack of unity in nursing? Can there be any unity if such diversity is accepted as the norm? Will members of the discipline be forced to travel forever on discrete trails on our discipline's journey, never to merge, never to converge? Sue Donaldson's and Hannah Dean's contributions lead us to the premise that such a conclusion, while possible, does not have to become a reality. Both of these authors noted that the discipline of nursing, as a practice discipline, is linked completely and absolutely to the recipients of our knowledge, that these recipients, through their societal mandate, justify the ongoing existence of any discipline. When and if a discipline fails that mandate, its own existence will be called into question.

Unity in and for nursing science then comes from society's mandate. This social mandate not only directs our discipline but also charges our diversity in that same direction. If nursing science is to meet its challenge, it will need many tools, tools that are best founded in our diversity. There may be schools of thought that do not serve in meeting our mandate or some aspect thereof, but we should not rush to abandon any school of thought until it can be clearly established that such a belief system makes no contribution to nursing's effort to meet its societal mandate.

Increasingly, the discipline has come to understand that the public mandate to nurses is the diagnosis and treatment of human responses to health (American Nurses' Association, 1980, 1994). This mandate can be met only through gaining the scientific knowledge that directs the nurse in caring for and treating human responses to health. Some of the knowledge required to treat these responses, especially those that are physiological, is best developed using empirical methods founded in the school of empiricist thought, whereas knowledge required for the care and treatment of psychological or social responses may best be developed within a postmodern belief system.

However, the development of our social mandate, the scientific and practice knowledge regarding the diagnosis and treatment of human responses, is a different journey. If we are to embark upon this journey, we must first understand the many pathways we will need to explore. We must come to understand the strengths and limitations of each belief system and where each school of thought will lead us in our science and our practice within society's mandate for the care and treatment of human responses to health.

References

American Nurses' Association. (1980). *Nursing: A social policy statement*. Kansas City, MO: Author.

American Nurses' Association. (1994). *Nursing: A nursing policy statement* (Revision/draft). Washington, DC: Author.

Index

Adorno, T., 206
Aesthetic criticism, 214
Analytic component, 16
Antirealists, 8
Applied science, 265, 267, 269
Awareness, 143

Bacon, Francis, 17
Being, 148
Belief system, androcentric, 128
Bias, 17
Bodies, 181, 182
Bottom line, 34

Caring, 171, 273, 280
Causal inference, 7
Causation, 9
Chaos theory, 14, 35
    deterministic randomness, 35
Client, autonomous perspective, 6
Client health, 4
Clinical tasks, 6
Cognitive authority, 54
Communicative action, 211, 217, 218, 222
Conceptual:
    activity, 67
    boundaries, 89

change, 82
    problems, 83
Conceptualization, verbal, 21
Concrete activity, 67
Consciousness, 142, 147
Consensus, 76
Consensus formation, 77
Context, 24, 165
    description, 24
    of discovery, 45
Critical theory, 61, 94, 205, 206, 207, 210,
    220
    Morrow, R., 221
Culture, 183

Deductive reasoning, 16, 17
Deductivism, 17
Deinstitutionalization, 248, 252, 254, 256
Descriptive studies, 15
Dewey, J., 29
Disciplinary matrix, 47, 63, 65, 67, 68
Discipline, 62, 63, 65, 66
    of nursing, 5, 81
    role of individuals, 84
Discourse:
    explicative, 214
    practical, 213
    theoretical, 213

Disembodiment, 198, 199
Doctoral degree programs, 4
Donaldson, S. K., 63, 279
Dualism, Cartesian, 200

Eidetic structures, 143
Emotions, 180
Empirical:
    knowledge, 64
    method, 109
    problems, 82
Empiricism, 2, 13, 15, 16, 17, 23, 25
    assumptions, 14
    contemporary view, 13
    paradigm, 236
    significance in nursing, 24
Enlightenment theories, 102
Epistemology, 110, 113
    definition, 113
    feminist, 114
    Marxist, 116
    nature of, 115
Equality of opportunities, 101
Ethical awareness, 194
Evaluation of theory, 79
Evolutionary, 59
    change, 73
    philosophy, 60
    school, 81, 82, 89
Exemplars, 48
Experience, intersubjective, 152
Experiment, 21
Experimental approach, 21
Experimental confirmation, 21

Facts, theory neutral, 7
Feminism, 61, 91, 93, 96, 97, 109
    methodologies, 95
    radical, 97
Feminist, 59
    approach, 137
    critique, 128
    epistemology, 105
    inquiry, 117, 118
    method, 91, 106, 108, 109, 125
    research, 114, 120, 121
Feyerabend, P., 94
Frankfurt School, 94

Freud, S., 188

Gender, 106, 117, 118, 121
Gender, activities, 107
Genealogy of problems, 84
Generalization, 8
Generative philosophy, 68, 69
Gilligan, C., 99

Habermas, J., 208, 210, 212, 218, 220, 223, 225
    methodology, 222
    theory of argumentation, 221
Hard science, 35
Heidegger, M., 140, 147, 148, 150, 157, 178
Heideggerian phenomenology, 8
Hermeneutics, 92, 185, 191, 196, 205, 223, 239
    of choice, 194, 198
    phenomenology, 149
Higher education, societal value, 3
Home care, 89
Horkheimer, M., 206
Human discernment, 195
Human experience, 182
Human misery, 5
Human responses, 23, 297
Human suffering, 10
Husserl, E., 140, 142, 143, 145, 147, 152, 156, 161
Hypotheses, 20
    alternative, 22

Intentional structure, 142
Interpretivism, 205
Intersubjectivity, 151
Intertheoretic reduction, 45
Interviewing, 165
Inward understanding, 85

James, W., 29, 32
    bottom line, 32
    value of ideas, 32
Justice ethic, 99

Knowledge:
    application of, 84
    clinical relevance, 66
    experience, and, 144
    nursing, 282
    objective, 140
    science, 157
    scientific, 140, 291
Knowledge generation, 60
Kockelmans, J. J., 188
Kuhn, T., 41, 43, 50, 51, 52, 53, 54, 60, 61,
        77, 79, 94, 112, 117
    mature science, 49
    progress in science, 52, 53
    scientific growth, 46
    view of science, 47

Laudan, L., 60, 61, 73, 74, 75, 77, 81, 82, 86
Levin, 182, 226
Lewis, C. I., 32
Lexicon, 48
Lived experience, 141, 144
Locke's theory, 20
Logical empiricists, 16
Logical positivism, 21, 27, 59, 60, 65, 94

Marcuse, H., 206
Marx, K., 188, 206
Matrix, 63
    disciplinary, 63
McClintock, B., 100
Medical intervention, 272
Mental disability, 245, 248, 249, 253, 255,
        258
Mental illness, 245, 250
Merleau-Ponty, M., 140, 142, 154, 155, 156
Method, 111, 112
    androcentric assumptions, 107
    critical theory, 224, 225
    disputes, 76
    empirical-analytic, 209
    experimental, 65
    feminist, 108, 121
    hermeneutic, 179
    Marxist, 108
    phenomenological, 159
    scientific, 93, 295
Model of care, practice partnership, 88

Models, deterministic, 18
Moral development theory, 99

National Institute for Nursing Research,
        85
Natural science research, imitation of
        research style, 107
Nature of reality, 34
Nature of scientific knowledge, 82
New knowledge, 229
Nightengale, F., 88, 89, 159, 195, 269
Nonquantitative variables, 34
Nurse:
    expert, 268
    interviewers, 162
    job satisfaction, 86
    scientists, 66
    societal commitment, 15
Nurse-patient relationship, 88
Nursing:
    academic, 277
    academic discipline, 276, 284
    actions, autonomous, 7
    administration, 82, 89
    alleviation of human misery, 5, 39
    applied science, 263, 273
    belief systems, 295
    caring practice, 263
    clinical practice, 291
    diagnosis, 285, 297
    discipline of, 295, 296
    doctoral education, 292, 293
    Hermeneutical approach, 176
    Hermeneutical model, 175
    knowledge, 205, 296
    philosophical foundation, 58
    philosophy of science, 59
    practice, 80, 264, 280
    practice discipline, 73
    practice, power, 243
    practice, scientific inquiry, 276
    practice, theory 216
    process, 285
    professional, 288
    professional identity, 275
    research, 284
    research in, 275
    science, 79, 278, 279, 295, 296
    science, pluralistic approach, 73

science, purpose, 15
science, society's mandate, 1
scientific identity, 288
societal mandate, 296, 297
study of human responses, 279
theory, 276
world view, 61
young science, 59

Objective knowledge, 44
Objectivity, 17
Observation, 20, 21
Ontological:
    convergence, 52
    definition, 35
    truths, 171
Operationalism, 27, 33, 34
    outcome measures, 37

Pain, 127, 130, 131, 137
    analgesic response, 136
    infants, 131
    management, 128
    medical management, 130
    narcotic administration, 131
    surgical management, 131
    unique to women, 133
    women, 133
Paradigm, 44, 47, 48
    acausal, 9
    conceptual clarity, 31
    crisis, 51
    incommensurability, 51
    lexicon, 47
    object domain, 51
    Peirce, C., 29, 30, 31
    signs, 31
Paradigmatic, 59
    view, 60
Perceived needs, 159
Perception, 156
Phenomena of interest, 77
Phenomenology, 92, 140, 141, 144, 145,
        154, 157, 239
    basic themes, 148
    clinical nursing, 160
    Husserlian, 179
    method, 155

reduction, 146
research, 172
Philosophers:
    poststructuralist, 239
Philosophical foundation, 58
Philosophy of science, 81
    generative, 61, 62
    nursing practice, 59
    postmodern, 91
Physicians, 95
Plurality of causation, 22
Popper, K., 16
Positivism, 16, 207
Postmodernism, 116
Poststructuralist, 9, 92, 234, 235, 244, 246
    analysis, 241, 243
    instruments of discipline, 237, 238
    power, 235, 236, 243
    science, 233, 239, 240, 241
    theory of, 242
Practice:
    discipline, 1, 5, 69, 285
    knowledge, 66
    science based, 5
Practitioners, 66
Pragmatic:
    approach, 79
    method, 28
    method, definitional clarity, 28
    process, 186
    theory, choas, 36
Pragmatism, 2, 7, 10, 11, 27, 94
    assumptions, 33
    central themes, 30
    conceptaul clarity, 30
    evolving movement, 29
    outcome variable, 28
    practical consequences, 30
    versus pragmatic, 38
Praxis, 54, 84, 85
Predictability, 14
Predictive knowledge, 208
Prescriptive theories, 1, 5
Probabilistic models, 19
Professional recognition, 291
Puzzle-solving, 55

Qualitative:
    paradigm, 10

science, 37
variables, 34

Racism, 121
Reality, 141
Received knowledge, 6
Reduction, 161
Related disciplines, 67
Research:
    critical action, 227, 229, 230
    phenomenology, 164
    poststructuralist, 234
Rogers, M., 188

Schiller, F. C. S., 29
Schutz, A., 140, 151, 152
Science, 62, 64, 93, 94
    aim, 62
    androcentric, 128
    clinical practice, 292
    communal activity, 54
    culture, Western, 95
    disagreements, 76
    evolutionary view, 41, 72
    feminist view, 72
    historical development, 81
    human, 266
    normal, 50, 54, 60
    paradigm bound, 50
    philosophical view, 43
    pluralistic view, 72
    prenormal science, 50
    rational problem-solving activity, 41
    revolutionary view, 44, 72
    traditional view, 72, 130
    value free, 45
    value judgements, 55
Scientific:
    inquiry, 121, 276
    knowledge, 84
    method, 110
    orthodoxy, 50
    problem, focus for scholarly acitivity,
        82
    progress, 10, 46, 75

rationality, 74
realism, 8, 9
revolution, 44, 50
Semantic empiricism, 27
Social:
    inquiry, 109
    processes, 109
    psychiatry, 226
    science, 154
    situation, 183
Societal value, practice of nursing, 4
Society, 62
Structuralist, perspective of science, 9
Substantiation, 19, 22

Themes, 168
Theoretical models, 18
Theorists, feminist, 104
Theory:
    feminist, 113
    problem-solving effectiveness, 75
Theory choice, 52
Therapeutic critique, 214
Thought, 150
    hermeneutic, 188
    knowledge, 139
Toulmin, S., 81, 82
Toulmin's model of evolutional
        conceptional change, 87
Traditional:
    research methods, 106
    science, 7, 8, 150
Traditional science, quantitative
        research, 8

Understanding, interpretation, 149

Vulnerability, 196, 197, 199

Women healers, 95
Women's movement, 106
World, spheres, 102

About the Contributors

Anne H. Bishop, Ed.D, M.N., R.N., is Professor of Nursing at Lynchburg College, where she teaches psychiatric-mental health nursing and a senior seminar that deals with philosophy, ethics, legalities of nursing, and trends and issues. She is currently Project Director of the Nursing Center for Health Promotion, which is supported by a grant from the Division of Nursing. Through the Center, faculty in the Department of Nursing at Lynchburg College are developing health education/health promotion teaching materials at a fourth-grade level to be used in conjunction with the programs for clients at the Free Clinic of Central Virginia. She has been recognized by her colleagues with the Outstanding Member Award of the Virginia Nurses' Association (1976) and the Nancy Vance Award (1990). She was selected as Outstanding Faculty Scholar at Lynchburg College in 1992. For 15 years, she and John R. Scudder, Jr. have been engaged in developing a philosophy of nursing that to date has produced four books: *Caring, Curing, Coping: Nurse, Physician, Patient Relationships* (Alabama, 1985), *Nursing: The Practical, Moral and Personal Sense Nursing* (SUNY, 1990), *Nursing: The Practice of Caring* (NLN, 1991), and a recently completed book on nursing ethics.

Evelyn Calvillo, D.N.Sc., R.N., was an Associate Professor in the School of Nursing at California State University, Los Angeles, at the time of her collaboration with Barbara Riegel and others on the chapter focusing on a generative philosophy of science.

Luther Christman, Ph.D., R.N., F.A.A.N., is Dean Emeritus of Rush University, President of Christman, Cornesky, and Associates, and an Adjunct Professor at Vanderbilt University.

Marlene Zichi Cohen, Ph.D., R.N., is Associate Professor and Director, Office of Nursing Research, University of Southern California, Department of Nursing, and USC/Norris Comprehensive Cancer Center, Los Angeles, California.

Hannah Dean, Ph.D., R.N., is Associate Chief of Nursing Service/ Research at the Veterans Administration Medical Center in Sepulveda, California. She has held faculty positions at California State University at Dominguez Hills, the University of North Dakota, Sonoma State University, and St. Xavier University. She was Director of the School of Nursing at Southern Oregon University in Ashland, Oregon, from 1985 to 1987.

Sue Karen Donaldson, Ph.D, R.N., F.A.A.N., is Dean of and Professor in the School of Nursing and Professor of Physiology in the School of Medicine at The Johns Hopkins University in Baltimore. She has held faculty positions in nursing and physiology at the University of Washington, Rush University in Chicago, and the University of Minnesota at Minneapolis. She occupied the first endowed chair for nursing research in the nation, the Cora Meidl Siehl Chair at the University of Minnesota. Her basic research is in the area of striated muscle physiology, and she established the multidisciplinary Research Center for Long Term Care of the Elderly in the School of Nursing at the University of Minnesota. She is an elected member of the American Academy of Nursing and the Institute of Medicine, National Academy of Science.

Laura Cox Dzurec, Ph.D., R.N., is an Associate Professor at the University of Maine in Orono and Clinical Specialist in Psychopharmacology Service at Acadia Hospital in Bangor, Maine.

Naiema Gaber Elsayed, Ph.D., R.N., is a faculty member of the School of Nursing at the University of Alexandria in Egypt.

Sara T. Fry, Ph.D., R.N., is Henry R. Luce Professor of Nursing Ethics at Boston College School of Nursing, where she teaches the philosophy of nursing, nursing ethics, and conducts clinical nursing research.

Ruth Ginzberg, Ph.D., is Assistant Professor in the Philosophy Department at Weslyan University in Middletown, Connecticut.

Sandra Harding, Ph.D., is Professor of Philosophy and Women's Studies at UCLA and the University of Delaware. She is author and editor of many books on science, epistemology, feminism, and postcolonialism, including *Whose Science? Whose Knowledge? Thinking From Women's Lives, The Science Question in Feminism, Feminism and Methodology, Sex and Scientific Inquiry,* and *The "Racial" Economy of Science: Towards a Democratic Future.*

Inger Margrethe Holter, Ph.D., R.N., is an Associate Professor at the University of Oslo, Institute for Nursing Science in Norway. She received the basic nursing education for diploma from Deaconess Hospital School of Nursing in Oslo and her M.S. and Ph.D. in nursing from the University of Rhode Island. She is author of several articles in English and Norwegian on critical philosophy and action research.

David L. Kahn, Ph.D., R.N., is an Assistant Professor and Luci Baines Johnson Fellow at the University of Texas at Austin School of Nursing.

Christine E. Kasper, Ph.D., R.N., F.A.A.N., is an Assistant Professor in the School of Nursing at the University of California at Los Angeles. Her research focuses on the effects of atrophy on skeletal muscle function and on the adaptation of skeletal muscle to microgravity environments, which has been studied during NASA shuttle missions. She has authored over 40 research publications in this area. The recipient of multiple grants from the National Institutes of Health, NASA, and the American Nurses' Foundation for studies in skeletal muscle physiology, she has been nationally honored for her research and work with students and has been elected a Fellow in the American Academy of Nursing.

Jacquelyn Ann K. Kegley, Ph.D., is CSU Outstanding Professor of Philosophy at California State University at Bakersfield.

Hesook Suzie Kim, Ph.D., R.N., is a Professor at the University of Rhode Island College of Nursing. She is author of a theoretical treatise, *The Nature of Theoretical Thinking in Nursing,* and has published several articles and book chapters on the nature of nursing knowledge development.

Patricia Lee, M.N., R.N., is a Family Nurse Practitioner at the Veterans Administration Medical Center in West Los Angeles and a doctoral student in the UCLA School of Nursing.

Carol Mack, M.N., R.N., is a doctoral student at UCLA School of Nursing.

Anna Omery, D.N.Sc., R.N., is Assistant Director of the Dumont-UCLA Transplant Center and Director, for Nursing and Clinical Research. She is an Assistant Clinical Professor at the UCLA School of Nursing. Her research focus is on bioethics and qualitative research, especially phenomenology. She continues to be an active participant in the debates regarding the philosophical foundations of and for the discipline of nursing.

Gayle Giboney Page, D.N.Sc., R.N., is an Assistant Professor of Nursing at Ohio State University. The focus of her program of research is the immune and metastatic consequences of postoperative pain. Throughout her clinical practice of caring for critically ill infants recovering from surgery, she has sought to deal with the many issues associated with attaining adequate pain control for these patients and to demonstrate that there is a biological consequence for experiencing unrelieved postoperative pain.

Francelyn Reeder, Ph.D., R.N., is an Associate Professor at the Center for Human Caring in the School of Nursing at the University of Colorado. She is author of several articles and book chapters on nursing science development.

Barbara Riegel, D.N.Sc., R.N., F.A.A.N., is Clinical Researcher and Coordinator in the Clinical Research Program at Sharp Memorial Hospital in San Diego.

John R. Scudder, Jr., Ph.D., is Professor of Philosophy at Lynchburg College in Lynchburg, Virginia. He began bringing his understanding of phenomenology and the human sciences, focused on history and education, to bear on nursing in the early 1980s when he and Anne Bishop began developing a philosophy of nursing. Their research to date has produced four books: *Caring, Curing, Coping: Nurse, Physician, Patient Relationships, The Practical, Moral, and Personal Sense of Nursing: A Phenomenological Philosophy of Practice,* and *Nursing: The Practice of Caring.* In 1986, he received both the T. A. Abbott Award for Faculty Excellence, given annually to one faculty member of the 17 colleges and universities related to the Disciples of Christ, and the Outstanding Faculty Scholar Award from Lynchburg College.

Pamela Shuler, D.N.Sc., R.N., is an Assistant Professor in the School of Nursing at the University of Kentucky in Hazard.

Bonnie Ellen Siegel, D.N.Sc., R.N., is a private consultant in nursing administration in Los Angeles.

Richard H. Steeves, Ph.D., R.N., is an Associate Professor in the School of Nursing at the University of Virginia.

Cathy Rodgers Ward, D.N.Sc.(C.), R.N., C.N.A.A., is Assistant Director of Nursing at the UCLA Medical Center and Assistant Clinical Professor in the UCLA School of Nursing.

Sandra J. Weiss, Ph.D., D.N.Sc., F.A.A.N., is a Professor in the School of Nursing at the University of California at San Francisco. She is currently Director of the Center for Family Health Studies and Chair of the Academic Senate for all sciences faculty at UCSF. She has received the UCSF Distinction in Teaching Award twice as well as the Helen Nahn Research Lecture Award. She has been actively involved with professional organizations, including the Governing Board of the American Academy of Nursing and the American Heart Association in San Francisco as both its Vice President for Research and Chair of the Board. Prior to coming to UCSF, she was Executive Director of the Health Care Consortium, a nonprofit research and educational institute.

Her scientific preparation is in two fields: child and family mental health nursing and biological and developmental psychology. Her program of research focuses on sensory vulnerability due to genetic predisposition or disease and the ways in which caregiving can influence health, development and recovery form illness through modulation of sensory stimulation. She has published extensively in this area, especially regarding measurement of interpersonal touch, vulnerability to touch, and the effects of touch on neurobehavioral response.

Printed in the United States
119738LV00002B/52-63/A